Second Edition

It's your Body...*Ask*

Your Guide to Talking with your Doctor about Breast Cancer

William H. Goodson III, M.D.

Fort Alexander Press

It's your Body...*Ask*

Your Guide to Talking with your Doctor about Breast Cancer

William H. Goodson III, M.D.

For leavy love —
With respect for his special efforts
to reduce cancer.
Best Regards
BN Gordon
2017

Dedicated to my patients, from whom I have learned

TABLE OF CONTENTS

PREFACE TO THE SECOND EDITION

Understanding what your doctor has found and what she or he proposes for you is the foundation for making informed decisions about your care. It is your right to know and to understand what your doctor is doing for you or, in the case of surgery or drugs, to you. Detailed medical terms are often unfamiliar, but most medical words can be explained using familiar terms. The purpose of this book is to help you understand the questions you can ask to understand the *words* your doctor is using.

Treatment of breast cancer has changed radically since I wrote the first edition of *It's your Body...Ask!* However, the questions to ask your physician have remained surprisingly similar. Where questions have changed it's because advances in treatment have made it relevant to ask new questions that would not have made sense before.

Sixteen years ago, breast oncology seemed to have arrived at a plateau. At that point in time, the general plan of therapy for breast cancer could be summarized in several pages and some key questions. Not any more!

Writing about breast cancer today, it isn't possible to provide answers that are certain not to shift in the next decade, or next year, or even next week. What is possible, and what I will attempt, is to provide an overview of how your physician thinks about your breast cancer, and how that understanding guides the choices that are available to you.

Treatment is still directed at 1) eliminating the cancer where it began in the breast, and 2) preventing or treating any cancer that might spread outside the breast.

A major shift in thinking has come about with the realization that there are more treatments that physicians can suggest than is always best or wise to do. Considering *how much to do instead of thinking about everything that could be done* began with the recognition that it was not helpful to remove the entire breast for most women with breast cancer. More recently we have learned most women can be adequately treated with removal of only a couple of axillary (armpit) lymph nodes —skipping the total node removal that used to be standard —and many women do not get enough benefit to justify chemotherapy or radiation therapy.

The second principle that has assumed greater importance is that the absolute benefit of therapy is always in proportion to the absolute risk. If the situation is challenging, a specific treatment may make a large absolute difference in what happens to a woman. However, if the cancer is less dangerous, the same treatment may make very little difference in what happens to a woman. Specifically, the less the risk, the less the absolute benefit of any treatment.

As before, this book introduces you to the questions that your physician considers as he or she recommends treatment. Ask your physician to help you understand what is the best and most current information now.

It's okay to ask. After all, it's your body.

PREFACE TO THE FIRST EDITION

Two comments as you begin this book: First, it is tricky to simplify anything as complicated as breast cancer. On the other hand, excessive detail can be extremely difficult to organize and to understand. For this reason, I have written in generalities on the assumption that a survey is the best way to begin. Second, this book, like all medical science, is a work in progress. Things change. For example, the two trials of post-mastectomy radiation mentioned in the book were not published until a year after the first draft was completed. And the Food and Drug Administration (FDA) approved HER2 antibody as a prognostic test for breast cancer while we were preparing the final draft.

Because this book is written in generalities, and because of change, no book will ever be the final authority. However, it can provide insight into how your doctor has been taught to think

Your decisions should be based on discussions with your physician. My hope is that this guide will help you with that conversation.

HOW TO USE THIS BOOK

Talking with your physician can be overwhelming if you are not accustomed to medical terminology. Doctors talk about unfamiliar ideas and provide a lot of information that is difficult to follow and to remember in an orderly fashion. However, if—*before you meet with your doctor*—you can anticipate what your doctor will talk about, the time with your doctor will be more productive.

The goal of *It's your Body...Ask* is to help you begin learning before you talk with your physician. This book does not replace your physician; your physician is always the best source of *personalized information* concerning your breast care. However, this book prepares you to ask the most important questions and to understand your physician's answers.

This book has an introduction and three sets of questions. The introduction will tell you how to get ready for the meeting with your physician. It explains where physicians get information and how to ask why your physician is recommending a specific action. It explains how to understand the statistics that your physician uses and will give to you. It suggests questions to ask yourself as you prepare to visit your doctor.

The main part of the book has three sets of questions. As you read through the main part of the book, you should focus on the section with questions that meet your needs (of course you can read them all if you prefer). The three sections are as follows:

Part One: Questions to ask if you are healthy but want to be certain that you have no signs of breast problems.

Part Two: Questions to ask if you or a medical specialist thinks you might have disease in your breast.

Part Three: Questions to ask if you have been told that you have breast cancer.

If you are facing a serious breast care problem such as cancer, you need information. Information, no matter how unpleasant, gives you power. When you know what your choices are, and the possible outcomes of each choice, you have the best opportunity to decide what choices you want to make.

Remember that no matter how dangerous a situation might seem, no one really knows what the future will hold for you. The best any physician can do is to tell you what has happened to women with similar conditions who were treated in the past. We never really know how new treatments will work in the future. And, we don't know the outcome of old treatments given to a person today until time has passed and we have the legacy of that experience.

INTRODUCTION:
PREPARING FOR THE APPOINTMENT WITH
YOUR PHYSICIAN

Where Physicians Get Information

There are four main types of information. Some are very reliable; others are less reliable. That is to say, you can put more faith in some types of recommendations than others. When your physician makes recommendations, ask what information she or he has used as the basis for the recommendations. The following are the questions to ask about different types of information.

"Are your recommendations based on medical tradition?"

There is nothing wrong with medical tradition, but it is only as strong as saying, "We always do it that way." Some traditions such as caring, confidentiality, or respect for privacy will probably never change (at least we all hope not). Other traditions should be challenged. An excellent example is the radical mastectomy, which was done by tradition for more than 80 years. Only when the tradition was challenged did we learn that often breast cancer can be treated without removing the entire breast.

"Are your recommendations based on personal experience?"

If you see a specialist who has seen many cases like yours, then her or his experience has some validity. However, you can understand how valuable your physician's experience will be for you only if you ask about that personal experience. Ask how many people your physician has seen who are like you.

If you have a rare condition or situation, then even a few similar patients in the past is relatively a lot. But if you have a common situation, you would not rely on your physician's personal experience unless she or he has seen many persons with similar situations.

If your physician is a generalist, or even a specialist, there are frequently better ways to make decisions and give you recommendations. Personal experience or traditions are appropriate bases when there are no other sources of information.

"Are your recommendations based on reports of the care of large numbers of women?"

Much better advice for you is based on a large past experience with women in similar situations. The way a physician gets access to broad experience is by reading many articles in which other physicians report their experience with similar groups of patients.

If your physician has published a formal article on a particular aspect of the information she or he is giving you, this will also be valuable, but only as a part of the published experience of other physicians who have also looked at similar groups of women.

Typically, a physician will publish an article about a group of women evaluated or treated in a certain way. Such a group of women is sometimes called a *series of patients* to indicate that they were a group of women treated serially, i.e., in the order they arrived, within a certain time period and in a certain way.

For most aspects of breast care, it is important to have enough patients in the series for it to be reliable. It is also important to have follow-up on such a group of women for a long enough time that you can reliably know what to expect, at least 5 and preferably 10 years from now.

"Are your recommendations based on a randomized clinical trial?"

A randomized clinical trial is the best way to compare two or more ways of diagnosing or treating breast conditions. It is impossible to compare two treatments if the women treated in each way were not similar before the treatments were given.

In a randomized clinical trial, similar women are divided into two groups. Each group is assigned to a different treatment. This division is not due to the choice of an advocate of one specific treatment, but by chance. In this way the groups of women are as similar as possible, and you can identify the effect of the treatment.

Randomization reduces bias from selection of women with less dangerous cancers for the physician's favorite treatment.

    (For further discussion of *bias*, see the next section on statistics.)

Key To Quality Of Information

In this book I will indicate the quality of information that is available to answer each question question using the key below:

Means randomized clinical trials.

Means observation for many years of what happened to large numbers of women treated in the past.

Means the personal experience of an expert in treating breast conditions.

Means medical tradition not supported by follow-up of large numbers patients or a randomized clinical trial.

At times I will give my own opinions. I will mark these with a ## unless there is significant published information to support my opinion.

In general it is best to use #### information and sometimes ### to make decisions. Use ## or # information only when other information is not available.

Understanding Statistics

    Statistics do not tell you what to do, but they give you information about what is more or less likely to happen if you make certain choices.

    Statistics are a way to learn from the experience of people who have had cancer or other questions about their breast care in the past. Statistics allow us to use that experience to estimate what will happen if you make different types of decisions. They are a way to explain to you the collected experiences of what happened to other people who started where you are and ended up in different directions. They are history.

Statistics estimate what is likely to happen.

    In a way, statistics are like a map or a chart of the ocean. They can tell you what is more likely to happen if you go in certain directions or make certain choices. Statistics cannot, however, tell you exactly what will happen. Just as in the middle of the ocean winds, tides, or storms can take you to a different place from where you intended, your experience with your health will not always be the same as that of other people. However, if you want to arrive at a specific destination, it is more likely you will arrive at that destination if you head in the right direction.

It is most common and easiest to understand statistics as a graph or line that shows what happened to many women in the past.

Imagine that 10 years ago, someone called a meeting of 100 women who had just been diagnosed with breast cancer. Suppose the same person took a photograph of this group of 100 women. Next, imagine that each year these same women were called together and a photograph of the group was taken again. It is the unfortunate truth that after a year there would be women who could not be in the picture because their cancer had progressed. Some would be sick and some would even have died.

Each year, the group in the picture would be different. You would celebrate the lives of those who were in the photograph. You would be sad for those who were not able to be there. You could also count the number of women who were in each picture and draw a graph that showed how many women were still healthy after 1, 2, 5, 10, or 20 years. This is what is done to create statistics. You count the number of women who have had different experiences.

Statistics are important for two reasons.

First, statistics are the best information available to a woman who has learned that she has breast cancer. They can give her an idea of what is likely to happen in the immediate future, and what might happen years later. When you look at a graph, it is important to understand that each point on the line represents women who were previously in some group years ago, and the graph tells what happened to them. It is important to remember, however, that *statistics are the history of other people* and that they never represent what will necessarily happen to you.

Second, statistics help a woman understand the outcome of her choice of treatment. For example, statistics tell that the number of women who will still be in the picture 10 years after a small breast cancer is virtually the same whether a woman has only the cancerous part of her breast removed or chooses to have her entire breast removed (see page 84). The same number of women will be in the group photograph. Statistics also tell us that, for women with certain types of breast cancer, treatment with drugs or hormones will make it possible for more women to continue to be in the photograph.

Statistics can also be subject to the bias or opinions of the people collecting the statistics.

For this reason there are mathematical tests of statistics and there are specific ways that statistics should be used to decide if one treatment is better or worse than another.

For example, physicians have learned over the years that some cancers will cause less trouble than others. A well-informed physician can select a group of women who will have a very high probability of survival, even if they have breast cancer. If a physician treats only very healthy women with very favorable cancers in a certain way, then the group picture of women with that treatment 10 years later will still show most of the women. The problem is that his information would not show that the treatment works. Rather, it would show that these women did well as a group. The physician knew from the beginning that the group of women would do well, and they would probably have done well *without* this treatment, too. This is biased patient selection.

Randomized Clinical Trials:

To avoid bias and make information more useful, physicians use *randomized clinical trials*. In a randomized trial, physicians gather a single group of women who have similar cancers. With these women's permission, they are assigned by chance (or, as physicians say, *randomly*) to one treatment or another. This is the only reliable way to compare two or more treatments.

It is important also to know that the predictive strength of statistics relies on the difference in the number of bad events rather than simply the size of the study. For example, if physicians compare results between two groups of a million women each, but only 10 women had a bad event—for example 2 in one group and 8 in another—it would not be meaningful since it would be such a small part of each group. At the other extreme, a study of two groups of 100 women each would be very meaningful if 20 women had a bad event in one group and 80 women had a bad event in another group. There must be many events to make useful comparisons.

It takes courage for a woman to enter a randomized clinical trial. Women who have breast cancer today owe a debt of gratitude to the thousands of women who agreed to participate in randomized clinical trials 20 or even 10 years ago when much less was known about the results of treating breast cancer.

Before You Go to Your Physician's Office

When you consult with your physician, it will be more productive if you decide in advance why the visit has been arranged. You may have different reasons at different times. However, the reason you are going to your physician will usually fall into one of three categories that you can identify by the topics listed below:

- "I am all right as far as I know, but I want an evaluation of my breasts." All the questions involving screening and general preventive measures will be discussed in Part One.

- "I have noticed something—or my physician, nurse, mammogram, lover, etc. has—and I am concerned about it." Most commonly, concern is caused by pain, a discharge, a possible lump or an area on a mammogram, ultra sound, or an MRI; but there are other causes for concern. The questions to ask will be discussed in Part Two. Specific concerns about your breast raise three additional questions: Does your physician agree that something exists? Is the finding a sign of cancer? If it is not cancer, what, if anything, is the appropriate treatment?

- "I have breast cancer and want to understand my options for treatment." Part Three will discuss what to ask when you know you have cancer.

Before you go to your appointment you should also gather all of the information that is available about you. This should include any images that have been made (usually available on a computer disc from your radiologist), biopsies, and the written report of the observations of previous physicians or other breast specialists such as specially trained nurses. Begin your appointment by telling your physician why you are there.

PART ONE

QUESTIONS TO ASK IF YOU ARE HEALTHY

You don't think you have a problem now, but you want to make informed decisions about your breast care. This section includes information on screening for breast cancer (clinical breast examination and mammograms), risk factors, and lifestyle issues.

"What is screening?

Screening is looking for cancer before it becomes so noticeable that it cannot be ignored.

One hundred years ago, breast cancer was usually diagnosed when a woman found a mass that caused an open sore, or was so big or so painful that it could not be ignored. The average size of breast cancer at diagnosis was four centimeters (a little less than two inches) and 90% of breast biopsies confirmed cancer. Starting around 1910 with Cancer Week in New York City, women were urged to be aware of their breasts. In the 1920s some physicians began to do breast examination for asymptomatic women, but it is instructive that a leading medical student textbook did not even mention breast examination until the 1942 edition.

The effect of increased awareness and breast examinations was that the average size of breast cancer at diagnosis dropped to about 2.5 centimeters (about one inch) by the 1950s. The down side of this was that only about 10 percent of breast biopsies were cancer. Ninety percent of biopsies could have been avoided if it had been known in advance if the lump was not cancer. Whether these were *unnecessary biopsies* is debated. A major issue is that neither clinical examination nor mammograms (that were introduced later) can prove that an area is cancer or not. Only a biopsy can determine whether an area is cancer.

Your opinion on the issue of knowing for certain is central to whether you will decide to request breast cancer screening for yourself.

"What is the benefit of screening?"

Survival is better when cancer is diagnosed at a smaller size as shown by the benefits of mammograms (discussed further below). And screening finds cancer at a smaller size so the surgery, when needed, is less complicated.

"What are the most recent breast cancer screening recommendations?"

The most recent recommendations at the time of this edition, written by an 11-person group sponsored by the American Cancer Society (ACS), were published in November, 2015. This guideline development group included four doctors who presumably have experience actually treating patients, two statisticians, two epidemiologists, two patient representatives, and *one economist*. The recommendations were published in November, 2015. The ACS previously published recommendations in 2003, and, although there is no announced schedule, it is likely that revised recommendations will be published in the future.

The 2015 ACS recommendations are only for *average risk women* (higher risk women are discussed later in this section) and rely exclusively on selective use of mammograms:

1. Women should be allowed to have screening mammograms between age 40 and 44 if they wish.
2. Women 45 to 54 years of age should have annual mammograms.
3. Women 55 years of age and older should transition to mammograms biennially (every two years) and continue as long as their life expectancy is 10 or more years.
4. Clinical breast examination is not recommended for average risk women of any age (please see discussion below).

"What are the theoretical harms of screening?"

In the lay press, it makes a "good" story to stir controversy, and this can be done easily by quoting persons who emphasize the so-called *harms* of screening. These so-called "harms" include financial and emotional costs. Whether you think these "harms" are important is a personal decision.

Screening costs money. First, there is the initial cost of taking and interpreting the mammogram (or clinical breast examination as discussed below). Second, there are costs to identify the reason that a mammogram or clinical breast examination is abnormal, in those cases where it is abnormal. These are the cost of additional mammograms, ultrasounds, and sometimes a biopsy. In some studies, if a woman has an annual mammogram for 10 or more years, there is a 60% chance she will be asked at least once to return for additional films. Because only about 10% of biopsies of palpable masses are cancer and about 20% of biopsies based on abnormal mammograms (without a lump) are cancer, the cost of a biopsy is "unnecessary" if cancer is not found. However, biopsies are only done when there is no other way to know if cancer is present.

Screening induces stress. As noted, up to 60% of women who have annual screening mammograms for 10 or more years will eventually have a mammogram that is called worrisome or incomplete by a radiologist. These women are usually asked to return for an ultrasound or additional mammograms of the area in question. For most of these women, a biopsy is not recommended, but they experience stress of worry about the possibility of having a biopsy.

Women who have a biopsy that does not find cancer undergo stress from the biopsy. They worry about the biopsy until the results arrive, and they may worry about their own future risk of cancer even if the biopsy is not cancer. If cancer is not found, the biopsy does not benefit a woman's health, and the stress would not have occurred if no one had suggested a biopsy. This stress lasts up to a year or longer in some studies.

It is argued that this stress is a "harm." *There are, however, no similar studies of stress for women who have skipped screening and then are found to have breast cancer that might have been found sooner or smaller.*

Cancers found by screening may never have grown enough to cause a problem. For nearly 40 years, some people have argued that screening identifies areas that look like cancer under a microscope but that would never have endangered a woman's health. It is unclear, however, at what point in the transition from being a very small area to becoming a large palpable mass these people would decide that a lesion is dangerous to a woman's health. The same people often assert that modern chemotherapy and hormone-based therapy are so effective that they compensate for delayed diagnosis, and early detection of breast cancer is no longer important. The average benefits of cancer drugs are indeed remarkable, but as discussed in the section on treatment, *they are not foolproof.*

There is a small physical risk from any biopsy. There is the risk of bleeding, infection, and a very small risk of complications of anesthesia, including an extremely tiny risk of death if a general anesthetic is used for the biopsy. However, virtually all biopsies can be done with local anesthesia, often with sedation, so the risk of long-term harm is extremely low.

"Who decides what screening to recommend?"

Screening recommendations are written by groups of people who read articles, interpret those articles, and write recommendations after discussing the relative harms versus benefits of screening. The writing groups consider the costs, possible benefits, the number of women who must be screened to save one life, the so-called harms listed above, and other factors related to their fields of training and their personal experiences. Writing groups are not infallible, and in many ways they are not without biases of their own. Their recommendations may fail to be logical, such as for breast examination discussed below.

Writing groups are sponsored by various organizations, for example, the American Cancer Society, the American College of Radiology, and the United States Preventive Services Task Force.

"How reliable are screening recommendations?"

Recommendations are only as useful as the data on which they are based, and whether the group asks the logical questions. For example, as discussed below, whether a clinician should examine the breasts of women without symptoms is not a simple issue of whether examinations can be proven to save lives.

Breast Examination

"Why would I request a breast exam from my doctor?"

Cancer can only be treated if you know it's there, and, as of 2016, clinical breast examination (CBE) has a role in identifying cancer. Mammograms miss about 15% of cancers. The 15% of breast cancers missed by mammograms is usually first identified by the patient or her physician feeling a mass or lump.

For women under age 50, over half of breast cancers are first identified as a palpable mass by the woman. Approximately one in eight breast cancers is first identified by clinical breast examination (CBE). However, a frequent scenario attributes diagnosis to a mammogram even when the first identification was as a mass. For example, a woman feels a mass and calls her doctor's office. The office refers her directly for a mammogram, and the mammogram confirms what the patient felt. It is said that the mammogram found the cancer, but the *initial identification* occurred when the patient felt a mass.

It is illogical when guidelines argue all three things, i.e., that physicians should not do breast exams *and* that women should not do self-examinations (discussed below) *and* that women under 45 should not have mammograms. Such guidelines would eliminate all three of these ways to find cancer. This kind of thinking would only make sense if breast cancer never occurred in women under age 45. Unfortunately, breast cancer does occur in women under 45 and leaving recognition of that cancer until it demands attention would be to step back 100 years in the care of breast cancer.

To avoid this logical dissonance, *it is my personal opinion that clinical breast examinations should be done on a routine basis.*

"What is the most important part of a breast examination?"

Very little is done to study breast examination because there is so much emphasis on mammography to compensate for short office appointments.

There are many components of an extensive breast examination that are taught to medical students. It turns out, however, that the most important part of a breast examination is palpation (feeling and touching) of a woman's breasts while she is lying on her back.

In a series of 1400 women diagnosed with breast cancer, only one cancer would have been missed if she had a mammogram and all the other steps of the clinical breast examination had been skipped *except palpation when the woman was lying down* ###.

Validating a shorter CBE is helpful because one of the reasons given to omit CBE is that many non-expert teachers have adopted a CBE technique that requires up to 5 minutes per breast to complete. In experienced hands, however, a good screening examination of palpating both a woman's breasts can be done in an average of 2 minutes ###.

The other important factor for a good clinical breast examination is that the clinician must actually pay attention to what she or he is doing.

"What does a basic screening examination feel like?"

A good clinical breast examination (CBE) is done by an unhurried, objective examiner. I use the word *examiner* because a specially trained nurse or other trained practitioner can do a good breast examination. The important point is that the person doing your examination should do many breast examinations on a routine basis.

To begin a screening CBE, you should be undressed sufficiently that both breasts can be seen and examined at the same time. During the examination, the examiner will usually spend at least a full minute palpating each breast. You should be aware that your physician is feeling your chest just below your collarbone, around to the side of your chest, and down to the line where a bra would lie below your breast. You should be aware that all of the area of your chest has been checked. This should include palpation of your nipple and areola, the softer area just around your nipple. The examiner will also palpate both breasts at the same time to check for symmetry. An experienced examiner can complete this palpation in an average of about two minutes.

"What is a detailed CBE?"

If you or your physician has noted a possible mass, if you have an abnormal mammogram, ultrasound or MRI, or if you have another breast symptom, a detailed CBE should be done. In that case, in addition to palpation just described:

• Your examiner should stand in front of you and look directly at your breasts. During this part of the examination, you should be asked to put your hands on your hips and push down or forward, to raise your arms, or to move your arms in some other way that causes your breasts to lift and pull up.

• Your examiner should feel under your arms and you should expect this to be a little uncomfortable.

• Your examiner should examine you while you are lying down as described above.

• Your examiner should palpate both breasts at the same time, with one hand on each breast, to check for symmetry.

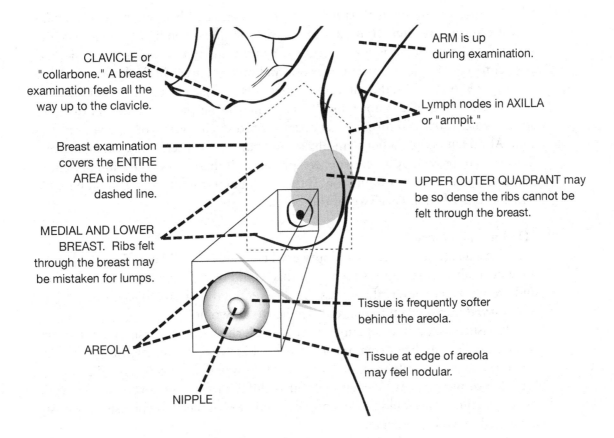

CLAVICLE or "collarbone." A breast examination feels all the way up to the clavicle.

ARM is up during examination.

Lymph nodes in AXILLA or "armpit."

Breast examination covers the ENTIRE AREA inside the dashed line.

UPPER OUTER QUADRANT may be so dense the ribs cannot be felt through the breast.

MEDIAL AND LOWER BREAST. Ribs felt through the breast may be mistaken for lumps.

Tissue is frequently softer behind the areola.

AREOLA

Tissue at edge of areola may feel nodular.

NIPPLE

These steps for your breast examination are the same ones that your physician has read about and has been taught. I describe them from your perspective because that way you can decide whether you have had an adequate examination.

"Did you find anything on my examination?"

After you are satisfied that you have had a good examination, the only other question is whether the examination found anything that was not typical.

It is a common misconception that women without cancer have "normal" breast examinations that do not find anything that is not typical of all women. Atypical areas are common (note: although the word *atypical* is used, this is *com-*

pletely unrelated to atypical tissue on a biopsy discussed below). In the Canadian Breast Cancer Screening Trials, about 7 to 8% of all women had an area that was not typical. However, it is not correct to say that this is a false positive CBE. It is correct to say that, if a clinician does not find unusual areas in the breast of about 1 of every 8 to 10 CBEs, the clinician is habitually doing a perfunctory examination.

If something that is not typical was found during the examination, the next steps should be decided through a cooperative process between you and your physician. Although people other than physicians can perform screening examinations, it is better to be seen by an experienced physician if there is any question of abnormality on your breast examination. If there is an abnormality, you should be evaluated as described in Part Two of this book.

"Do I need a biopsy?"

The exception to needing a biopsy is when there is a valid question of whether an abnormality exists. It may seem that this would be a simple question to answer, and often it is. However, all women are different and there really is no such thing as a *normal* breast examination that applies to all women.

Breasts develop in too many different sizes, shapes, and consistencies to have one particular way be normal for all women. Likewise, if your breast is different, that does not necessarily mean it is abnormal. As noted, in screening studies, about 7 to 8% of women have something that is different from the average ###. Your breast examination should make sense in the context of the many breasts previously examined by your physician.

Sometimes your physician may suggest a recheck of a given area within 8 to 12 weeks. At the end of that time, however, either everything should seem very much as expected, or further evaluation is appropriate ###.

Mammograms

"Do I need a mammogram?"

Routine mammograms look for areas in your breast that might be cancer. A mammogram does not diagnose cancer, and a negative mammogram does not mean that there is no cancer. A mammogram is only a test that looks for areas that might be cancer. Mammograms can miss cancer!

On the other hand, mammograms can find the signs of cancer before you or your physician's examination can feel the cancer. Frequently the cancers found by mammograms are smaller than those found by examination. Randomized clinical trials, in which women were or were not asked to have routine mammograms, recorded fewer deaths from breast cancer among the women who were having routine mammograms ####.

For women over 50, it is generally agreed that mammograms can change the course of cancer by early detection. Thus, women over 50 should have mammograms every year or at least every two years. Note that all of the randomized studies of mammograms separated women according to age, not whether they had gone through menopause. Studies were done with women over 50 and, in one study, over 55. When these studies started, most women had gone through menopause by age 50, so these age numbers were chosen as a *simple* way to separate women into pre- and post-menopausal groups for the purposes of the studies. Since the 1990s many women go through menopause after age 50. Whether mammograms are more effective after age 50, or after menopause, or after both is not actually answered by any study.

For women younger than 50, the randomized trials have not demonstrated as much benefit from early detection through mammography. Using a statistical method called meta-analysis that combines many studies into one report—and in this case excluding results from one large study that disagreed with their conclusions—some researchers have concluded that mammograms do not have significant benefits in women under 50. However, recent long-term (20-year) follow-up from one of the largest studies has still shown a benefit for women who started mammograms at age 40 ####.

Part of the controversy arises because there are fewer women who develop breast cancer before age 50, so more mammograms must be done to find the number of cancers that must be studied to show the same benefit (remember that the strength of statistics is determined by the number of adverse events—such as having cancer or death—not simply by the number of women in each group page 19). And there are plausible explanations for the less-clear benefit in younger women. The breasts of women younger than 50 tend to be denser (see page 43 for more about breast density), and mammograms do not work as well in dense breasts. Also, women younger than 50 are often preoccupied with work, children, or their own parents and will sometimes ignore a lump if they have the reassurance of a negative mammogram. Remember, however, that at least a fifth of invasive cancers in young women are not detected on routine mammograms.

Mammograms do benefit some women younger than 50, and there are many stories of women younger than 50 whose cancer could not be felt but was found by a mammogram. The important point is to realize that mammograms are more likely to be inaccurate in women younger than 50 than in women older than 50.

"Why do the newest recommendations recommend starting mammograms at age 45?"

It is a simple matter of dividing the women between 40 and 49 years of age into two groups. There are fewer women who develop breast cancer between 40 and 44 years of age (0.6%) than between 45 and 49 years of age (0.9%). (The sum of these risks is the 1.5% on page 39.) Thus, more women will need to be screened to find one cancer.

Guidelines do recommend screening starting at age 40 for higher-risk women. However, breast density on a mammogram can only be identified with mammography (see below) and mammographic density is a risk factor in its own right.

"Why do the new guidelines recommend two years between mammograms after age 55?"

In addition to reviewing randomized and un-randomized trials of screening, the ACS guideline-writing group commissioned the Breast Cancer Surveillance Consortium (BCSC) to look at their data for differences between breast cancers found with mammograms once a year versus cancers found with mammograms once every two years (biennially). The BCSC is a group that records data on mammograms from several screening centers in the San Francisco, California, Bay Area.

For *premenopausal women,* the BCSC found that mammograms once a year identified *smaller and less dangerous cancers than with screening every two years.* Thus annual mammograms are recommended for premenopausal women.

For postmenopausal women, there was no average difference in the tumors for women—without other risk factors—who had screening every two years compared to once a year. Note that the similarity of outcomes with different screening intervals is not according to age, but rather according to *whether a woman has gone through menopause.* Given the number of women who menstruate well past age

50, it is important to personalize the age at which even to consider less frequent mammograms *for average risk women.*

The BCSC writers acknowledged that this is an observational study, not a prospective trial. An accompanying editorial comments, "The frequency of screening mammography should be *personalized based on risks,* such as breast density [discussed below], age, family history of breast cancer, and history of breast biopsy. Depending on age, menopausal status, and other risk factors, some women may need to opt for more frequent mammograms and others for less frequent screening."

The best way to decide what to do for a woman who has passed through menopause may be to consider her personal factors. If she has dense breasts on mammograms she may consider continuing mammograms annually until her breasts become less dense. If she has other risk factors, she may consider continuing annual mammograms. If, however, she has less dense breasts and she does not want to do annual mammograms, there is support for spacing her screening mammograms to once every two years.

"Why do the guidelines recommend screening as long as a women has 10 year life expectancy?"

It takes approximately 10 years from the time of screening to find a survival benefit from screening. Thus, as long as a woman has at least a 10-year life expectancy, she will be likely to benefit from screening mammograms. If, however, a woman has significant heart disease, lung disease, kidney disease, or other chronic illness, there is a real risk that any kind of treatment will make her health worse, and she is unlikely to gain a survival benefit.

"Can't I just have a breast exam?"

Results of the Canadian Breast Cancer Screening Trial have been used to suggest that clinical breast examination (the longer examination described above) is as effective as mammograms to find cancer ####. This study has two limitations: First, the mammograms were not up to current quality standards, i.e., they took only one image of each breast instead of two, the machines were not up to current standards, and most important, the mammograms were not read by radiologists with special training in mammography. Second, the breast examination in this study was an intensive examination that required about 5 minutes to examine each breast for a total of 10 minutes palpating each woman's breasts. There is no trial to show that 10 minutes provides the best exam, and some experts think that a 2-minute exam is sufficient to decide if it is a normal result ##. In practice, the typical breast exam is so much shorter than even 2 minutes that conclusions from the Canadian Screening Trial cannot apply unless there is general conversion to using much more careful breast examinations.

"Is the radiation in the mammogram dangerous?"

There is no such thing as a totally safe dose of radiation, although recent work suggests that very small doses spread out over time are less risky than the same doses in a short time. We know from studies of women exposed to radiation at Hiroshima and Nagasaki, as well as other intentional uses of medical X-rays, that radiation can cause breast cancer. Therefore, the question is not whether the mammogram is safe, but, rather, what is the risk of the mammogram versus the possible benefit of finding breast cancer with a mammogram before the cancer can be felt.

In a simplified analysis of the worst-case scenario, it is estimated that mammograms might cause cancer in about 1 woman of 10,000.

In this same group of women, about 10% (or 1,000) will develop cancer after age 45. About 20% of these (or 200) will die of breast cancer.

Early detection with mammograms will reduce cancer deaths by about 30%; stated another way, approximately 60 women will have a life benefit from the mammogram. Sixty chances to avoid death from breast cancer constitute a greater possible benefit than the one chance to cause cancer.

The discussion is actually more complicated, however, because (as discussed before) the clearest benefit from mammography is in women over 50, and studies of women over 50 are the universally accepted basis of saying that mammography will reduce breast cancer deaths.

Further, it is younger women, especially those younger than 30, who are most susceptible to radiation causing breast cancer, and the benefits of mammography are less clear for younger women. Thus, mammography is a fairly straightforward trade-off of a smaller risk for a greater benefit for a woman over 50; but the benefits versus risk are less clear for women under 50 who are presumably pre-menopausal. (Remember that this refers to routine screening mammograms only.)

There is no way to avoid one or the other of these risks. You will either choose to have a mammogram or choose not to have it, but choosing not to have a mammogram will not take away your risk of having breast cancer. It is simply a fact to consider that 1 woman of 10,000 might have a cancer caused by the mammograms and die from it, while approximately 60 additional women of that same 10,000 will survive a breast cancer that otherwise would have been fatal.

Another way to think about mammograms:

It may be simpler if you think of this as two possible groups you might join, each with 10,000 women.

The first group has no mammograms. About 1,000 women will develop breast cancer and about 200 women will die from breast cancer in this group. There is no way to know if you are a woman in that group who will die. You know only the chances for the group as a whole.

If you join the second group of women who have mammograms, about 1,001 women will develop breast cancer (the 1,000 expected plus the 1 extra breast cancer), but only about 140 will die from it. There is a slightly increased risk of developing breast cancer with the mammograms and radiation, but a big decrease in the risk of dying from breast cancer.

Your physician will have thought these ideas through and will probably recommend the mammogram if you are over 50. If you are under 50, you should discuss the risks versus the benefits with your physician. The choice, however, is yours.

"Is my mammogram being done correctly?"

A mammogram is more complex than it would seem at first thought. A good mammogram requires a sharp image of the largest portion of your breast possible.

The American College of Radiology has a special training program to certify that mammograms are made in the optimal way. This means that the radiologist is qualified, the technicians are qualified, and the machines are calibrated on a routine schedule to be certain you don't get more X-rays than are necessary. It is best to have your mammograms done in a center that has been certified by the American College of Radiology.

When you make a mammogram appointment, ask if the center uses a dedicated mammography machine and whether the American College of Radiology certifies the center. If the answer to either of these is *no,* go to another center.

As with your physical examination, you should notice certain things while your mammogram is being taken:

- The machine should be one that is used only to take mammograms and it should be calibrated at regular intervals to be certain that the dose of radiation you receive is the smallest possible. It is easy and appropriate to ask the technician, casually, if the machine has been calibrated recently. If it has been done, the technician will usually respond with reassurance. If there is a sultry reply, ask exactly when it was last calibrated. Machines should be calibrated at least every month, but to insure accuracy a weekly calibration is preferable, and many centers calibrate daily.
- The technician should ask you if there are any areas of concern so that she can focus extra attention on those areas.
- The technician should draw your breast into position on the machine when she prepares to take your films; often it will feel like your breast is being pulled forward. If the technician takes a picture of only the part of your breast that easily falls onto the X-ray machine, she will be missing a significant part of the breast where cancer can begin.
- The technician should compress your breast in the machine. It will be uncomfortable, but if there is not squeezing, the picture will show tissue gathered into clumps that could be mistaken for masses. When compression is used properly, the individual parts of the breast are gently spread apart so that each area can be viewed individually.
- The technician should ask you to hold your breath while the picture is taken. The mammogram is taken very quickly, but if you're breathing, the picture might be blurred. Blurred mammogram pictures make it particularly difficult to find calcifications, which are the first sign of many cancers.

"What is 3-D mammography or tomosynthesis?"

Standard two-dimensional (2D) mammograms use two images of each breast. Each picture shows the sum of all tissue in the breast.

For tomosynthesis or 3D mammography, part of the machine moves, allowing a computer to create images of the breast as though it was many different layers. The radiologist sees the breast not as one mass of tissue, but as though they could flip through individual layers.

In early studies, tomosynthesis has been more sensitive and found more cancers than standard 2D images. Equally important, tomosynthesis is less likely to raise concern that a benign area might have cancer, which means that women need fewer extra studies to determine if cancer is present.

There is not yet a good comparison of 3D mammograms to MRI for women at high risk. With current systems, there is more radiation exposure with a 3D mammogram. Research is underway to improve the picture-taking process, reduce radiation, and to determine exactly how best to use 3D mammograms.

"Can't I just have an ultrasound?"

Ultrasound (or sonography) is the use of sound waves to study the density of tissue in different areas of your breast. This machine does not use radiation to study your breast. Instead, it uses very high-pitched sound waves that bounce off the tissue in your breast. The machine can tell what tissue is denser by the way the sound waves bounce back from inside your breast. Ultrasound can also identify fluid, provided the fluid has no debris in it.

Cancer is typically so dense that it reflects sound from its surface, but it reflects little or no sound from inside compared to normal breast tissue. The effect is that cancers often look dark on the screen because they do not reflect sound waves inside. Fluid-filled cysts, which are usually benign, can also look dark because the fluid does not reflect sound inside either.

The major limitation of ultrasound is that it cannot see micro-calcifications, which are one of the earliest signs of cancer seen on mammograms. If you omit mammograms in favor of ultrasound, you reduce the possibility of early identification of the two-thirds of cancers that have calcifications. Another limitation of sonograms is that they can study only a very tiny area of your breast at one time, so each part of the breast must be individually studied. Ultrasound also has more false positive examinations than mammography.

Ultrasound is useful for evaluation of a specific problem found on physical examination, a mammogram, or an MRI (see below), but less useful for screening the entire breast to discover if there is an abnormality. It is easy to miss small areas on sonography. A sonogram that shows signs of cancer will be very useful, but a negative sonogram, like a negative mammogram, is not useful to rule out cancer.

If there is a mass on a mammogram, the ability of a sonogram to identify a cyst is sufficient so that if the area is identified as a cyst, no further surgery or biopsy is needed. If, however, the area is solid, then some sort of biopsy is needed (see Part Two).

In general, mammography is still a better screening test, although ultrasound has become very useful. An ultrasound may be useful if your breasts are so dense that the radiologist cannot obtain a satisfactory mammogram and tomosynthesis is not available.

"Should I have an MRI?"

Magnetic resonance imaging (MRI) makes images without radiation. However, it is so sensitive that it finds many more things that are not cancer than do mammograms, i.e., it is less specific. Thus, MRI is not a good screening tool except for high-risk patients (see below).

MRI itself does not show cancer. It only shows the shape of breast tissue. An MRI study actually depends on two MRIs taken back-to-back. The first MRI shows the shape of the tissue in the breast. Between the two MRIs, the patient is given a drug, gadolinium, that makes blood look different. Then a second MRI is taken to identify areas that have more blood in them. These areas are said to *enhance*. Areas with cancer have more blood flow and will enhance on an MRI.

Because of its low specificity (many false positives), MRI screening is recommended only for women who have a high risk of cancer. Most insurance companies will approve MRI when a woman has at least a 20% lifetime risk of breast cancer. The clearest high-risk groups are women who have increased risk because of gene mutations such as *BRCA1* or *2, PALB2*, etc.

MRI can be used to evaluate the extent of cancer in the breast after a biopsy has shown cancer, but routine MRI before treatment is controversial. Sometimes your physician can persuade your insurance company to authorize an MRI to help understand a complicated problem such as discharge, unexplained persistent pain, or large cysts that are too numerous to count.

"What does the Bi-Rads score mean on my mammogram report?"

Radiologists use a score from zero to six to summarize their overall impression of a mammogram. This is the BiRads score, Breast Imaging Reporting and Data System:

Bi-Rads 0 There is a technical problem and the mammogram study is incomplete.

Bi-Rads 1 The mammograms are totally normal.

Bi-Rads 2 Finding that is definitely benign, e.g. scar from a previous biopsy.

Bi-Rads 3 Finding that is probably benign, but should be rechecked in 6 months.

Bi-Rads 4 Suspicious for cancer.

Bi-Rads 5 Almost certainly cancer.

Bi-Rads 6 Biopsy has already proven cancer exists and this is just checking for other areas.

Breast Self-Examination

"Will breast self-examination (BSE) help me?"

The answer is complex: "No: and "Yes." For this reason, breast self-examination (BSE) is—and will probably remain—controversial. The problem is that BSE was accepted as a good technique before any evaluation of its real effectiveness.

BSE is simple and practicing BSE does not directly add to health care costs, so many hoped it would help save lives. There are certainly many women who have practiced breast self-examination. Many women have found their own cancers earlier than if they had waited for a routine mammogram. Women who have learned BSE tend to notice cancers earlier. On average, they find cancers that are about 2.0 centimeters in diameter compared to about a 2.4-cm diameter for women who do not practice BSE and find their tumors by accident. The smaller size of cancers found by BSE is a fact, but that *does not prove that BSE saves lives.*

The World Health Organization sponsored two studies of BSE, one in the former Soviet Union and one in China, both where women had not heard of breast self-examination. Women with cancer were treated using Western standards. In both studies, women who were instructed in BSE found more cancers themselves. A higher percentage of women using BSE had smaller cancers and they could have breast-conserving surgery combined with radiation therapy for the treatment of their cancer. But, even after 10 years, *neither study* has shown that women who found their cancer with BSE live longer ####.

These results with BSE are very different from results of the studies of mammograms, where three major studies found improved survival from breast cancer by as soon as 7 years after the beginning of mammography.

The difference between mammograms and BSE is that mammograms can find smaller cancers that cannot be felt. A woman is more likely to benefit from early detection with a mammogram of a cancer that is too small to be felt than when the cancer is found with BSE. With BSE, even though it is found earlier, it is still large enough to be felt.

The clearest benefit of BSE is that if cancer develops, it is usually found in a smaller size and it can be treated with less surgery. Also, BSE or clinical breast examination by a physician or other examiner is the only way that about 20% of invasive cancers are found, especially in younger women ###.

"How should I do BSE?"

Your breast self-examination should mimic the examination your physician has given you. There are three keys to adequate BSE: familiarity, pattern, and palpation.

It is unlikely you have examined many women, but you compensate by being especially familiar with yourself. If you are going to do BSE, do it regularly but no more often than once a month. The best time is about a week after the first day of your menstrual period, if you are still menstruating, or on the same day each month if you are not.

If you find yourself rechecking an area, have this area evaluated by a trained professional. No one makes a truly objective evaluation of herself, and no one should have to make that kind of decision about herself.

The pattern you use to move your hand over your breast must take into account that breast cancer can start anywhere that there is breast gland tissue. Breast gland tissue can be anywhere from your collarbone to your lower chest and from one side of your chest to the other. The round protruding part of your breast—the part you think of as your breast—is often shaped as much by fat as by the breast gland tissue. If cancer exists, it starts in the gland tissue and can be in areas other than just the round protruding part.

You should pay close attention to the whole area of your chest (see page 28). Studies that have measured the percentage of the breast that women actually checked on BSE have found that it is best to use a pattern that ignores the nipple as the center of your breast. If you try to ignore your nipple as the center of your breast, you are more likely to feel the whole breast gland area.

For palpation, use three fingers at a time. Palpate with gentle circles feeling with the pulp or the fingerprint part of your fingers. This is the most sensitive part of your fingers and it will be most sensitive to any changes.

Risk Factors

"What is the average risk of getting invasive breast cancer?"
The risk of getting breast cancer during any specific year in your life is small. However, a total of about 12.5% of women in America will develop breast cancer if they live to age 85. This is the total risk over an entire lifetime when looked at from a young age.

These are average the risks of breast cancer in the next 10 years for a woman at different times in her life, based on U.S. government statistics updated in 2009:

Between ages 20 and 30, less than 0.1%
Between ages 30 and 40, 0.5%
Between ages 40 and 50, 1.5%
Between ages 50 and 60, 2.4%
Between ages 60 and 70, 3.5%
Between ages 70 and 80, 3.8%
Between ages 80 and 90, 3%

But it's important to look at what happens to a woman's risk of breast cancer during the rest of her life, starting at different ages:

Starting at age 20, the risk for the rest of her life is 12.5%
Starting at age 30, the risk for the rest of her life is 12.5%
Starting at age 40, the risk for the rest of her life is 12.4%
Starting at age 50, the risk for the rest of her life is 11.2%
Starting at age 60, the risk for the rest of her life is 9.4%
Starting at age 70, the risk for the rest of her life is 6.7%
Starting at age 80, the risk for the rest of her life is 3.8%

The risk drops with age because by the time a woman has reached 60, for example, she has *lived through some of her total risk*, and there is less time for her to develop cancer in her remaining lifetime.

The chance that a woman will die of breast cancer is much less than half of the chance that she will develop breast cancer. Specifically, in the same way that the lifetime risk of breast cancer is 12.5%, the lifetime risk of dying of breast cancer is less than 3%. Breast cancer is the cause of death for about 4% of the women who die each year in the United States, and breast cancer is the leading cause of cancer death for women between 35 and 50 years of age.

"Am I at high risk for breast cancer?"

Risk is defined in two ways: relative risk and absolute risk. Relative risk is the term more commonly used term by physicians, but it also is more easily misunderstood. It is it used so often—and it is so prone to misinterpretation—that it is worth a moment to explain the difference between relative risk and absolute risk. The other reason to understand the difference is that the same terms are used to describe the benefits of drugs to treat cancer.

Relative risk

Relative risk compares the risk of the study population to the risk of the general population. For example, women who drink two to three drinks of alcohol per day have about a 14 to 15% risk of developing breast cancer. The general population has about a 12 to 12.5% risk of developing breast cancer. The risk of 14 to 15% divided by the general risk of 12% gives a ratio of 1.2 (14.5% divided by 12% = 1.2). This is the risk of the study population (people who drink alcohol) *relative to the general population*. Thus it is risk of one group *relative* to another so 1.2 is called the *relative risk*.

Some researchers say that two to three drinks of alcohol per day is associated with a 20% increase in the risk of breast cancer. It is true that there is a 20% increase in the relative risk (1.2 is 20% more than 1.0), but this is often misunderstood to mean that one-fifth (or 20%) of women who drink this much will develop breast cancer, which is definitely not the case.

Absolute risk

Absolute risk is a term that most people can understand intuitively. It means the actual increase as numbers, as opposed to a proportion. For the example of women—of average risk—who drink two to three drinks of alcohol per day, the absolute increase in risk is 2.5%.

The term is called "Absolute Risk," but it is more intuitive to realize that it is really the absolute difference between two levels of risk. In the example of alcohol, the absolute difference in risk is only 2.5%—the difference between 12% and 14.5%.

When doing research, it is easier to calculate relative risk. Measurement of absolute risk means that women must be followed for longer periods of time.

"Does a biopsy showing atypical hyperplasia mean I have an increased risk for getting cancer?"

Atypical hyperplasia (discussed further on page 68) is a finding on a breast biopsy in which breast cells have started to grow in a specific abnormal way. This atypia can only be found by a pathologist looking at a tissue sample under a microscope. Atypia may initially be felt as a mass or seen as an abnormality on a mammogram, but it cannot be diagnosed by either a mammogram or palpation.

A woman with atypical hyperplasia on a biopsy has a relative risk of breast cancer of about 3.5 to 5. This means that her risk for the next 20 years is at least 3.5 times greater than that of the general population ###.

Since this diagnosis is often made in women in their 40s, the appropriate comparison is women of the same age. About 3% to 4% of women without atypical hyperplasia would develop breast cancer in the next 20 years. Three percent to 4% times 3.5 (the relative risk) is about 15%. Thus, 15% is the absolute risk that a woman with atypical hyperplasia will develop breast cancer in the 20 years after a breast biopsy with that diagnosis.

In general, most risk factors are useful for the scientific study of breast cancer, but they have very limited meaning for an individual woman. Relative risk for most risk factors, other than for atypical hyperplasia, family history, or a harmful gene mutation, is much less likely to have any impact on your life.

"What does it mean if I'm notified by my radiologist that I have dense breasts?"

To begin, studies of breast density *only apply to density on a mammogram*! There is a big distinction between breasts that feel dense on physical examination and breasts that look dense on a mammogram, because a breast can feel dense but be non-dense on a mammogram. What your breasts feel like does not predict the way they look on a mammogram. Only density on a mammogram predicts risk of breast cancer.

Radiologists use four categories to describe mammographic density:

- Extremely Dense is the most-dense category.
- Heterogeneoulsy Dense means the breasts have lost some density, but this is still above-average density.
- Scattered Densities (or Scattered *Fibroglandular* Densities) means the breasts have lost a lot of their density. When discussing risk, Scattered Densities indicates less-dense breasts and less risk.
- Mostly Fatty Replaced means most of the gland tissue has been replaced by fatty tissue. This is the least density possible.

"What causes breast density?"

Breast density is not a thing that a woman acquires in her life. *Density is natural situation that persists in some women*, but not in others. Almost all young women have dense breasts on mammograms. As women get older, some women's breasts become less dense while other women's breasts will stay dense.

The factors that determine why breasts stay dense are not fully understood, but women whose breasts stay dense are more likely to develop breast cancer.

"If I have dense breasts, how much risk does that indicate?"

The association of density and breast cancer is true ###, but it is important to put it in perspective. The way to do this is to think about the difference between relative risk and absolute risk discussed above with risk factors in general. It is true that women with extremely dense breasts do have about four times the risk of women who have breasts that are mostly fatty, i.e., with extremely low density breasts. However, *these extreme groups together are only about 10% of all women. The majority of women have either heterogeneously dense breasts or breasts with scattered densities.* The difference in these groups is only about twofold, and the line between these two groups is the average risk for women that specific age.

For example, if women of a certain age have an average risk of about 3%, a woman with heterogeneously dense breasts will have a risk of about 4% and a woman with scattered densities will have a risk of about 2%. The absolute difference between most higher-risk women and most lower-risk women would be only

2%, even though 4% is twice the risk of 2%.

Breast density can also categorize women with family history or a previous biopsy into higher or lower risk groups, but again the absolute differences are more meaningful than relative risk.

Breast density has limitations in its implications for individual women. Your physician can access a free, on-line calculator from the Breast Cancer Surveillance Consortium (BCSC) to personalize your risk for the next ten years. The Gail Model is a similar calculator that includes different factors such as age of first period and age of first full-term pregnancy that are not included in the BCSC risk calculator. The Gail model does not consider breast density.

Genetic Testing

"Will genetic testing help me know if I am at high risk?"

Genetic testing has changed the way physicians counsel women who have a family history of breast cancer. It is now understood that there are a small number of women with a family history of breast cancer who have also inherited a mutation in the *BRCA1* or 2 gene that predisposes them to a very high risk of developing breast cancer. Early studies, in highly selected families, suggested that up to 85% of women with mutations to the breast and ovarian cancer susceptibility gene (*BRCA*) would develop breast cancer; but fortunately, some recent studies looking at populations have found that the risk may be less than that for many women.

Either breast or ovarian cancer at a young age, in large numbers or across several generations—in either the father's or the mother's family—suggests that a family might have an inherited gene mutation. There are other women without a family history who might also consider genetic testing because studies find they might have a breast cancer gene mutation even in the absence of a family history. Therefore, genetic testing is recommended for anyone who develops breast cancer under age 50, women with triple negative breast cancer who are under 60 (discussed in Section Three of this book), women with two separate breast cancers (often but not always in different breasts), a woman who herself or whose relative has ovarian cancer, and any man with breast cancer.

BRCA1 and 2 were the first genes that were tested widely. PALB2, a gene necessary for the normal function of BRCA 2, is found in similar families. It is common to test genes in panels of 20 or more genes. There are some gene mutations that clearly predispose to cancer, but there are other mutations—called *variations of unknown significance* (VUSs)—that cannot be interpreted with current information. Some of these mutations do not change gene function, but some eventually are found to cause cancer.

Because of this increasing complexity, it is desirable to work with a trained genetic counselor to decide what genes to test and how to interpret tests. Responsible use of genetic testing involves informed consent and is provided by a specially trained genetic counselor who explains to a woman, before the tests, the emotional, legal, and medical implications of genetic testing.

"If I have a family history, but test negative for a gene mutation, am I still at high risk?"

Gene testing is primarily useful in two situations: if it is positive for gene mutation, or if a woman tests negative for a *specific mutation known to be present in a blood relative who has breast cancer.*

When a blood relative with breast cancer has tested positive for a gene mutation, that mutation probably explains the family history. Because the family history has been explained by the mutation, if a woman tests negative for that mutation, her risk is lower—but even then, it is still slightly above average.

In contrast, if a woman has a high-risk family—but no one with cancer has tested positive for a gene mutation—there is only a small likelihood, less than 20% in some studies, that she will have a gene mutation known to be associated with breast cancer. Nevertheless, these women are at increased risk of developing breast cancer even if they test negative for a mutation.

There is not an exact correlation between the results of genetic testing and a person's risk of getting breast cancer. That's because there are causes of breast cancer (environmental factors, for example) that are still not completely understood.

"Are there other gene mutations that increase the risk of breast cancer?"

A recent review identified 11 known gene mutations that are believed to increase the risk of breast cancer. The incidence of the BRCA genes is small except in families with a strong history of breast and/or ovarian cancer. The other gene mutations are rare even in families with a lot of breast cancer.

These genes—with their associated estimates of lifetime risk up to age 80—are as follows:

Mutations encountered in a moderate number of high-risk families

BRCA1	75% lifetime risk
BRCA2	76% lifetime risk

Mutations that are risky but generally very rare even in high-risk families

TP53 (or P53 mutations)	High but no reliable estimate of lifetime risk
PTEN	High but no reliable estimate of lifetime risk
CDH1	53% lifetime risk
STK11	High but no reliable estimate of lifetime risk
PALB2	45% lifetime risk
CHEK2	29% lifetime risk
ATM	27% lifetime risk
NF1	26% lifetime risk
NBN	23% lifetime risk

High-Risk Guidelines

"If I am at high risk, what can I do about it?"

There is no foolproof way to prevent breast cancer in women who are at increased risk. Surgery and drugs have been proposed, but both have risks as well as possible benefits, and neither has been shown to reduce risk without significant side effects. Surgery and drugs both attempt to reduce the risk of breast cancer by decreasing the amount of gland tissue in the breast that might eventually develop into breast cancer.

"Should I have my breasts removed before I get cancer?"

Surgery to reduce risk consists of removal of as much noncancerous, normal gland tissue from the breast as is possible. This is called a *prophylactic mastectomy*. Drug therapy suppresses growth of breast tissue and causes its involution. Involution is the normal process of aging in which the gland tissue of the breast dies for lack of hormones to stimulate its continued growth.

Although prophylactic mastectomy, removal of the breast tissue with or without removal of the nipple, has been proposed to prevent the development of breast cancer, there is no prospectively planned study of this attempt to prevent breast cancer. Two studies have reported unplanned series of patients ###.

Physicians at the Mayo Clinic studied 203 families in which they thought women had a high risk of breast cancer, either because there were multiple cases of breast cancer within the same family or because there were combinations of breast and ovarian cancer within the same family. In these 203 families, 214 women chose to have prophylactic mastectomies. These 214 women had 403 sisters who chose not to have mastectomies.

When the Mayo Clinic followed the 403 sisters who did not have prophylactic mastectomies, 38 developed breast cancer. Among the 214 women who chose prophylactic mastectomies, only three women developed breast cancer. When they made mathematical allowances for the length of time the women were followed, they estimated that prophylactic mastectomies reduced the risk of breast cancer by 90% and the risk of dying of breast cancer by 80%.

The reason cancer can still occur is that, as discussed under breast examination and BSE, breast tissue can exist anywhere from the collarbone to the chest wall below your bra line. Complete removal of all breast tissue would require removing all the skin in this area, which would cause unacceptable disfigurement. Even the most meticulous surgeon can remove no more than 90% to 95% of breast tissue.

"Should I take a drug to prevent breast cancer?"

Two kinds of drugs have been used to reduce breast cancer: drugs that modify the estrogen response (tamoxifen and raloxifene) and drugs that block formation of estrogens in the body (aromatase inhibitors).

In the NSABP-P01, the first trial ever to prevent breast cancer, tamoxifen caused a 45% reduction in development of breast cancer in a high-risk group of women. Although 45% is a correct description of the relative reduction in risk, the absolute reduction in breast cancer was 1.03%: from 2.3% in the placebo group to 1.27% in the tamoxifen groups. The 1.03% is 45% of 2.3%, but you get a more accurate idea when it's described in absolute terms: Tamoxifen prevents breast cancer in 1.03% of women who take the drug ####. Tamoxifen has not yet led to a reduction in death from breast cancer.

The argument against tamoxifen is that prolonged use of the drug is associated with a small, but real, possibility of causing cancer of the uterus in about 1 out of every 100 women. Tamoxifen is also associated with cataracts and with blood clots in the legs. For a woman *who has cancer* the benefits greatly outweigh these side effects, making tamoxifen the safest drug available *to treat breast cancer.* However, for woman without cancer these may be unacceptable risks relative to her absolute chance of getting breast cancer. Tamoxifen is good for your bones and your heart.

Despite these misgivings, it is exciting that any drug might change anything about the occurrence of breast cancer; and it is not impossible that tamoxifen might be reasonable for certain very high-risk people. If the risk of adverse side effects is always the same, tamoxifen might have a benefit that outweighed the risks for selected, very high-risk women. An example might be a woman with an inherited *BRCA1* or *BRCA2* mutation. Such a woman's lifetime risk of breast cancer is greater than 50% and accumulates at about 10% every 10 years. A 45% relative reduction in risk would equal an absolute benefit of a 5% decrease in the likelihood of breast cancer over 10 years. It might be reasonable to accept a 1% risk of tamoxifen's causing a uterine cancer if one had a real decrease of 5% in the risk of breast cancer.

Raloxifene has been tested against tamoxifen, but the results are only partially the same ####. Like tamoxifen, raloxifene reduces invasive breast cancer, but it does not reduce non-invasive breast cancer as well as tamoxifen. It still has the risk of blood clots, and like tamoxifen it is good for your bones and your heart. The surprise is that unlike tamoxifen, raloxifene decreases rather than increases the risk of uterine cancer. Unfortunately, raloxifene does not work to *treat* breast cancer.

Aromatase inhibitors (AIs) work by stopping the body from making any estrogen. Even after menopause, women make estrogens in fatty tissues, and make small amounts locally right in the breast. AIs eliminate this last bit of estrogen formation.

AIs reduce the risk of breast cancer more effectively than tamoxifen ####, but there are other limitations. AIs can stimulate the ovaries, so *they cannot be used in women who still have functioning ovaries.* AIs reduce the risk of uterine cancer, but they also make osteoporosis and heart disease more likely. They are used to reduce risk of breast cancer in women who have gone through menopause.

"If I am at high risk, should I have more breast imaging?"

Mammograms, beginning at age 40, are recommended for all women with a family history of breast cancer. If the relative with breast cancer was diagnosed when she was younger than 50, mammograms are sometimes recommended beginning at an age 10 years younger than the age at which the cancer was diagnosed.

For example, if a woman's mother was diagnosed at age 42, then mammograms for the woman would begin at age 32.

When there is a BRCA 1 or 2 gene mutation, or another gene mutation associated with high risk, MRIs are used in addition to mammograms and physical examination.

Screening with MRI, breast exams, and mammograms is recommended starting in the 20s for a woman who has tested positive for a personal gene mutation such as BRCA 1 or 2.

"Will I reduce my risk of breast cancer if I change what I eat or drink?"

Information about how your diet affects your chance of getting breast cancer is disappointingly limited.

Japanese women living in Japan and eating a traditional diet have a much lower rate of breast cancer than Caucasian women in the United States. Japanese women who move to the United States experience a higher risk. If a woman is of Japanese ancestry but grows up eating an American diet, she has a risk similar to a Caucasian American woman. It is often assumed that changes in diet explain these changes in breast cancer risk.

Obese women are more prone to breast cancer than non-obese women. Some results suggest that this does not apply to women who are obese from a young age. Rather, the effects of obesity are greater in women who become obese later in life, usually during mid-life.

Alcoholic women have more breast cancer than nonalcoholic women. Two or more drinks per day will increase the risk of breast cancer. In one study, an average of three-and-a-half drinks of alcohol per week increased the risk of breast cancer (a drink is defined as 12 ounces of beer, 3.5 ounces of wine, or 1.5 ounces of hard liquor).

A high-fat diet has been associated with breast cancer in some studies but not others.

The largest randomized trial showed a trend toward less breast cancer with a low fat diet, but did not reach the usual criteria to say it was a statistically significant difference. However, the study may have failed to show a difference because many women assigned to the control group, i.e., to eat their usual diet, changed to a low fat diet anyway. In the interest of your general health, it is probably best to limit fat in your diet. Of course, this is almost a prerequisite for avoiding obesity.

In other studies, eating cruciferous vegetables (broccoli, cauliflower, Brussels sprouts) may be helpful. If you like vegetables, these are a reasonable addition to your diet. However, the preventive effect of these dietary suggestions is small enough that if you do develop breast cancer it is not right to blame yourself for eating the wrong foods.

Studies of specific vitamin supplements have been disappointing, and at least one study shows that high doses of vitamin A or vitamin E can increase the risk of lung cancer in smokers.

"Will I reduce my risk if I exercise?"

Exercise reduces the risk of breast cancer, if you exercise to at least a minimum level. The minimum exercise needed to reduce cancer is at least 500 and probably closer to 1000 MET minutes each week ###. *MET* is an acronym for *Metabolic Equivalent of Task,* and it is used to compare the energy needed to perform different tasks. One MET is the energy to sit in a chair. Brisk walking, for example, uses three-and-a-half times as much energy as sitting, so it is 3.5 METs. One hour of brisk walking uses 210 MET minutes (60 minutes x 3.5 METs = 210 MET minutes). At this rate, it takes about 3.5 hours of brisk walking each week to get the health benefits of exercise from 500 to 1000 MET minutes.

More intense exercise uses energy faster, so the METs of running, for example, are higher. Thus, it does not take as long to use 500 or 1000 MET minutes of energy. For reference, 3.5 METs of brisk walking is fast enough that you cannot have a serious conversation, but slow enough that you can talk casually.

"Are plastics or other chemicals dangerous?"

There is an ongoing debate as to whether environmental exposure to bisphenol-A (BPA) in bottles, cans, or cash register receipts contributes to breast cancer. The same can be said of two other classes of chemicals, phthalates (THAL-ates) and parabens (PAR-a-bens), that are found widely in personal care products such as makeup, skin creams, shampoo, etc. We are exposed to these chemicals and many others every day.

Three things are definitely true: First, we know these chemicals are in our bodies because we can measure them coming out in urine, and both BPA and parabens have been found in breast ducts and breast tissue respectively. Second, if non-cancerous breast cells are exposed to these chemicals in a laboratory culture, the cells develop traits like cancer. Third, virtually all safety testing for chemicals has been done only for one chemical at a time, but we live in a "chemical soup" every day, and research is desperately needed to understand how mixtures of small amounts of many chemicals might add up to affect human biology more than a small amount of only one chemical.

For reasons that are argued by some to be reasonable—and thought by others to be inappropriately influenced by the chemical industry—there has been relatively little money available for research to determine the actual facts.

At the present, none of us can avoid exposure to environmental chemicals. However, *for myself*, I avoid canned foods when possible, I consult the website of The Environmental Working Group (see resource page), for names of personal care products with lower levels of suspect chemicals, and I do not heat food in plastic containers.

"Can I take birth control pills?"

Birth control pills are not associated with an increased incidence of breast cancer in women who have had children or who are older than 20 when they begin taking them ###.

The first oral contraceptives used in the 1960s had high doses of estrogen and have been shown to be associated with an increased incidence of breast cancer before the age of 30. It is not clear if this means that more women developed breast cancer or if these women would have developed cancer anyway, but the pill accelerated the cancer, causing the cancer to begin earlier. Today, oral contraceptives have a much lower dose of estrogen and, therefore, are probably safer.

A legitimate question remains concerning the safety of birth control pills for adolescents. Some recent studies show that younger women might increase their risk of breast cancer if they use oral contraceptives. Although, there is controversy about the objectivity of these studies, it is not accurate to say that oral contraceptives are totally safe in very young women.

The mitigating fact, *even for adolescents*, is that *oral contraceptives reduce the risk of ovarian cancer ###*. Moreover, they reduce the risk of ovarian cancer more than any possibly-observed increase in breast cancer. This also seems to be true for women with BRCA 1 or 2 mutations.

"If I used fertility drugs to have a baby, am I at higher risk?"

There have been questions of whether in vitro fertility treatment might lead to increased breast cancer in the mother. A recent study in the Netherlands did not find increased breast cancer in 25,000 women who had ovary stimulation as part of fertility treatment ###. If there is an increase, it is very small.

Hormone Replacement

"Can I take hormone replacement at menopause without increasing my risk of breast cancer?"

For years there were multiple studies looking at the use of hormones by women at menopause. In general they all found some increased risk of breast cancer in women who use hormones longer than 8 to 10 years, but the increase was minimal. The largest studies were the Nurses' Study and epidemiological studies done with follow-ups of other people. The remaining question was whether benefits in reducing heart disease would justify the small increase in risk of breast cancer. The Women's Health Initiative (WHI) was a randomized, placebo-controlled trial intended to determine the balance of harms versus benefits from hormone replacement therapy (HRT).

The WHI was actually two trials, one for women with an intact uterus, and one for women whose uterus had been removed by hysterectomy. Since estrogens given alone (like tamoxifen) increase the risk of uterine cancer, women with an intact uterus received progesterone with the estrogen because progesterone offsets or counteracts the effects of estrogen by itself on the uterus. Women who did not have a uterus did not need to worry about uterine cancer, so they received estrogen alone.

To everyone's surprise, the effects on the breast were opposite in the two trials!

Women who received the combination of estrogen and progesterone developed 8 more breast cancers per 10,000 person years. Think of that as 8 per 1,000 women followed for 10 years, which is about 0.8% more breast cancer after 10 years of combination (estrogen plus progesterone) HRT ####.

The surprise was that *women who received estrogen alone had 6 fewer breast cancers* per 10,000 patient years, or about 0.6% less breast cancer at 10 years ####.

The WHI studies were not stopped because of breast cancer findings. Instead they were stopped because of a parallel increase in the risk of stroke and heart disease. The major criticism of these studies, however, is that the average age of women beginning the study was 65. Older women may already have established blood vessel disease that can cause heart attack and stroke. There is follow-up data suggesting that if hormones are started within a few years of menopause, there will not be an increased risk of heart attack and stroke.

"Can men get breast cancer?"

Yes. Men can get breast cancer. Breast cancer is less common in men than is women, i.e., less than one percent of breast cancer is in men. However, breast cancer is increasing in men in the same proportion as it is increasing in women. Men have the same increase as women even though men don't take hormones at menopause, don't delay childbirth, don't take birth control pills, don't decide not to nurse their babies, and don't get over-diagnosed by mammograms. The similarity of the increased breast cancer in men and women raises the question of what environmental exposures they have in common.

"Are men with breast cancer treated the same as women?"

Yes. Breast cancer in men is usually like breast cancer in postmenopausal women, and it is treated the same. The questions in Section Two and Section Three of this book apply in almost the same ways to men as to women.

PART TWO

QUESTIONS TO ASK IF YOU HAVE
AN AREA OF CONCERN

Suspicious Areas

"Do I have a lump or other suspicious area?"

The answer to this question should be a simple *Yes* or *No*.

By definition, any lump or any other irregularity in your breast is suspicious. There is no manual test, physical examination, or mammogram that can tell whether an area in your breast is cancer. The only security you can have in examination is the observation by an experienced clinician that your breasts feel typical for a woman with your breast size, your weight, and your life history related to your breasts. This is not perfect, but it is all that can be done with an examination.

Any area that is not consistent with the typical palpation of breasts must be evaluated further. Only your physician can tell whether there is an area present that is not typical or as expected. If such an area exists, it demands further explanation.

The basis for understanding whether an area in your breast is unusual or atypical is to recognize that breasts have a typical structure. Different areas of the breast usually feel different, and some lumpiness can be typical in a given area of breast.

For example, the area in the upper part of the breast toward the armpit or axilla is often more dense than the other breast tissue. The area behind the areola (the darker skin around the nipple) is softer, and the edge of tissue around the areola is lumpy in many women. The area in the lower part of the breast toward the middle of your chest is likely to feel lumpier (see page 29). If you are large breasted, there may be a thickened area of tissue along the lower edge of your breast. Individuals may vary from these patterns and still be quite normal, but women who have different patterns of tissue should be checked very carefully for symmetry.

Events in your life have a major effect on your breasts. If your breasts were bigger at one time because of pregnancy, birth control pills, or weight gain, but now are smaller, they will often feel lumpier. This is not disease and it is not, as some physicians say, fibrocystic disease. It is the normal expected outcome of your life history. A scar can leave either a soft area where tissue has been removed, or it may be harder where the scar has formed. Changes after surgery are quite variable. If you have had breast surgery, you should ask your physician to help you understand what your breasts will feel like after the operation.

The main point is that, although breasts are all very different, they do follow typical patterns for the position of tissue, for areas that feel lumpier, and for areas of relative density. An experienced clinician will examine your breasts and determine whether they seem to be typical, taking into account both the variation among women and the tendency for all women to have fairly symmetric breasts.

You do not want your breast examiner to attempt to diagnose your breasts by what is felt. If your examiner says that she or he feels a lump but that it is OK and not to worry, demand more evaluation. Palpation is only about 70% reliable to decide if something is cancer or not. You deserve better.

"What does my physician or examiner mean if she or he says that an area is fibrocystic?"

Fibrocystic is a term used in three different contexts with three different meanings. Because it is not specific, the word *fibrocystic* has little real usefulness. You should be aware that *fibrocystic* has no agreed, uniform, or meaningful definition except as the specific result of a biopsy based on the removal of tissue from your breast.

The only consistent use of the word fibrocystic is by pathologists who use the term *fibrocystic condition* (NOTE: not fibrocystic disease) to describe certain changes in a woman's breast tissue that are seen on a biopsy and are not cancer.

Radiologists sometimes used this word in the past, but this is not advisable, since it has no real clinical meaning.

Unfortunately, physicians and other examiners often use the word fibrocystic to describe what they feel on examination, but there is no consistent definition of what constitutes a fibrocystic breast or area of a breast. Also, the term *fibrocystic* based on clinical examination has no relationship to development of cancer in the future.

"Will a mammogram help diagnose *the lump that I feel?*"

Mammograms can be useful, but they can also be very misleading, especially if you have found a lump.

If you feel an area, but the same area feels normal to your physician, it may be that you are sensitive to a change in your body that your physician cannot feel. A mammogram is sometimes useful to help your physician focus on one area and possibly select an area that should have a biopsy. If the mammogram is negative, however, you should continue with observation over time (as discussed below) rather than being reassured that what you feel is nothing.

Examination and mammograms together are very good to detect cancer, but they are not a complete evaluation. If they are negative, a repeat examination after 8 to 12 weeks, to be certain your breast examination is stable, is an important part of completing your evaluation.

A mammogram can be very misleading, especially if you and your physician rely on a negative mammogram to decide that something you feel is OK. Mammograms can be wrong! If there is any question in your mind at all, ask your physician to reexamine you after a short time.

"How can I find out what caused an area the radiologist spotted on my mammogram?"

A mammogram can tell whether there are areas that are not symmetric, whether there are areas that have changed between now and a previous mammogram, or whether there are obvious signs of cancer. The appropriate next step always depends on your personal situation.

If an area of your breast has changed, then your physician should have the same level of suspicion as if there were a specific sign of cancer. In general, your breasts should not change; if they do there must be an explanation.

If there is an area that is suspicious for cancer, then a biopsy is indicated. A needle biopsy may be useful; but if there is a suspicious area and a needle biopsy is negative, then a surgical biopsy is necessary.

Asymmetry is a more common finding and one that may be clarified by obtaining several opinions. In general, if there is an area of asymmetry on a mammogram, if there is no mass on ultrasound, and there is no palpable area on physical examination, then repeat mammograms can be used to follow the area. Experience has shown that asymmetry on a mammogram is not uncommon, just as asymmetry on physical examination is not uncommon. If asymmetry is stable over a minimum of two years of observation, then a biopsy is not usually indicated ###.

If there is an area of concern on your mammogram, you need an examination by a physician. It is best if your physician examines you before she or he looks at your mammograms. That way she or he can decide what is felt without having the mammogram suggest a finding.

If a questionable area is seen on your mammogram and this area is not palpable, then special techniques are needed that combine imaging (mammography, ultrasound, or MRI) with biopsy techniques. Sometimes the radiologist who does the imaging will perform the biopsy using a computer or ultrasound-guided technique. Sometimes the radiologist will place a mark (usually a wire) in the area where the mammogram shows an abnormality in your breast. In this second situation, your surgeon will use the wire as a guide to find the right area to biopsy. (See discussion of biopsies page 62.)

Breast Discharge

"Is it normal to have breast discharge?"

Breasts do not usually leak fluid. It is unusual to have spots of fluid appear on your clothes. However, if you squeeze your breasts or otherwise manipulate them (as with intimate relationships), it is not uncommon for normal breasts to have some fluid come from the nipple.

"Should I worry about my breast discharge?"

The majority of discharges are not indicative of cancer. Equally important, the majority of cancers do not have a discharge. There is only a weak relationship between cancer and discharge. The type of discharge determines whether you should be concerned. Although any spontaneous discharge can be associated with cancer, the most typical discharge with cancer is clear.

It is not necessary to squeeze your breast to look for fluid. If you squeeze your breast and obtain fluid, the fluid will often look black or very dark green. This is a typical color for fluid from the breast of a woman who is not nursing.

Normal women have fluid in their breasts during the reproductive years of their lives, so a discharge that comes only when you squeeze your breast is likely benign. It is there because the purpose of the breast is to make fluid (i.e., milk) when a mother nurses a baby. Squeezing simply pushes this fluid out where you can see it.

The majority of Caucasian women who are in the reproductive years of their lives will have fluid if they squeeze their breasts. Just less than a majority of African American women can express fluid, and about a quarter of Asian women can. These discharges reflect the natural function of the breast when normal hormones are present.

If fluid comes from your breast spontaneously, i.e., if spots of fluid or blood show up on your bra, nightclothes, or a towel after a bath, you should consult your physician. Although most of the reasons for spontaneous nipple discharge are benign, they should all be evaluated to rule out cancer. The scariest discharges are those with blood, but except for older women, these are less likely to be related to cancer.

Bloody discharge often occurs with a small tumor called a papilloma. Papillomas are not cancer, but they cannot be reliably diagnosed by imaging. Recent work suggests that if a biopsy shows a papilloma *without atypia*, the chance of cancer is low. If a papilloma has atypia, like all atypical lesions, it should be removed.

Bloody discharge can occur during pregnancy. The rapid breast growth during pregnancy will often create small irregular fragments of tissue within the breast ducts. These fragments of tissue look like papillomas under the microscope, but they do not become cancer. A bloody discharge during pregnancy usually stops when a mother starts to nurse, and unless there is a lot of blood, a biopsy is not necessary.

Breast Pain

"Should I be concerned about the pains I feel in my breast?"

Pain is unlikely to mean cancer: Very few breast cancers cause pain, and breast cancer is an uncommon cause of pain. Nevertheless, pain is never normal, although breast discomfort is typical in some situations. Likewise, the threshold where discomfort becomes pain is different for every person. Your physician will want to know when (time of day, time of month, etc.) you have pain, what makes the pain worse, how long you have had pain, and where the pain is located.

What you feel as pain has two components: 1) the sensation that is carried to the brain by nerves, and 2) the meaning that you attach to the sensation that your brain receives. Meaning is very important. For example, from infancy we have many sensations in different parts of our bodies that occur so often that we learn to experience them as normal. The breast is one of the places where these sensations occur. During adolescence you experienced many sensations including the normal feelings of your breasts. These feelings will always be there if you pay attention to them.

If a woman has a cause to worry about her breasts, she will sometimes notice sensations in her breast that she would usually overlook. It is not, however, appropriate to ignore pain without a thorough evaluation. It is useful for you to ask yourself whether the sensations you notice started in your breast, or if you have been made more aware of your breasts by some other concern.

The skin of your breasts is very sensitive, and light touch, sharp points, or hot or cold will be felt very acutely. The deeper parts of your breasts, however, are more sensitive to stretching. Stretching occurs when any tissue in your breast is pulled or made acutely larger.

If you are still having periods, your doctor will ask whether your pain changes at different times of your monthly menstrual cycle. The most common breast pain is related to changes in your breast that occur with the normal rise and fall of blood hormones. Late in your menstrual cycle, just before your period, hormones make your breast grow a little in many widespread parts of your breast. Each area that grows stretches a little and has sensations from that stretching. Any one of these points would probably be insignificant and unnoticed by itself. When your hormones rise, however, there are so many different areas of your breasts involved that all of these sensations together may be felt as pain.

Pain associated with hormonal changes has two very specific characteristics. First, it is diffuse in both breasts and it is worse either midway between two periods or just before your period. Second, it decreases or goes away after your period starts. Pain that is not like this cannot be diagnosed as simply related to menstrual cycle changes.

If you have gone through menopause and are taking hormone replacement therapy (estrogens, etc.), these medicines may also make your breasts grow. For this reason, you may have discomfort or occasional pain in your breasts. Like menstrual cycle changes, this pain is typically diffuse and will clearly start and stop when you take the medication or stop it for a while. (See Part One for discussion of whether hormones increase your chance of getting breast cancer.)

"What does it mean if I have pain in just one spot?"

Pain in just one area of your breast may be related to a mass, an infection, a solitary cyst, or rarely, cancer. It may also be related to monthly hormonal changes, but your physician will be able to ascertain this only after a careful evaluation. Also, in situations where cancer is a cause of pain, it is possible that the pain can be present before any lump is found on examination or any change is noted on a mammogram. The most your physician can do to evaluate the reason for your pain is a good physical examination and a mammogram, but you should expect that your doctor will be careful and recheck you in 8 to 12 weeks if the pain continues. MRI can sometimes be helpful.

Sometimes a pain continues in one place and there is nothing your physician can see, feel, or detect on a mammogram, ultrasound, or MRI. You can always feel the spot because it is within you; but unless there is an area your physician can localize, there is no foolproof way to rule out cancer. If there is nothing the physician can see or feel, there is no way he or she can know until a biopsy is done on the area you feel. Such cases are unlikely to be cancer, but the only way to be certain is to check the area every few months until either something becomes apparent or nothing becomes apparent after many months. It may also be useful to have another physician examine your breasts for a second opinion.

"Do we need to treat the pain in my breasts?"

Two issues arise in deciding to treat breast pain: Is the pain a sign of cancer, and how bad is the pain?

Pain is rarely a sign of cancer. Your physician should examine you and obtain mammograms. If your physical examination and mammogram are as expected for a woman your age and with your life history, you are probably safer if you rely on these and do not insist that your physician tell you what is causing the pain. Otherwise your physician may be tempted to classify your pain as "fibrocystic."

This may sound contradictory—that uncertainty is safer—but when there is no *certain* diagnosis, everyone, your physician included, will remain more alert.

There is no agreed, correct way to proceed in such situations. Speaking for myself, I sometimes tell a patient that I don't know for certain why she has pain. I can make up an answer, but then we will both be lulled by a false sense of security. Something that has a name will seem less dangerous or perhaps even be assumed to be safe. It is better to remain vigilant. When other tests fail, or cannot be applied, the best *test* is observation over time. If you push your physician into making a diagnosis, you will reduce the likelihood that observation over time will find something that might be important. It is hard to wait, but it is worse to jump to a conclusion that is misleading.

"What can I do about the pains I get in my breasts?"

If physical examination or mammograms reveal any new findings, they should be biopsied or treated specifically. If the results of the physical examination or mammograms are within normal range, decisions are more complicated.

Direct treatment of diffuse breast pain requires difficult choices. The drugs available to treat breast pain are effective, but they also have significant side effects. Bromocriptine causes nausea and headaches in many women, and danazol causes weight gain, irregular periods, and occasional masculinization such as facial hair. Tamoxifen has also been used for breast pain because it reduces the effects of hormones. These drugs work, but you must decide whether the pain is severe enough that you will accept the side effects.

Reducing the salt in your diet before your period starts is sometimes helpful. The hormones that rise in your blood before your period cause your body to retain salt, as well as causing growth in your breasts and uterus. Salt in turn causes your body to retain water, and the extra water will contribute to pre-menstrual weight gain, swelling of your breasts, stretching of breast tissue, and thus, pain in your breasts. Approximately 70% of women with normal periods experience some range of monthly discomfort in their breasts on this basis.

Evening primrose oil may help relieve pain in some women. The effectiveness has been tried in limited prospective trials, but some physicians are critical of the trials in the belief that they were not well done. On the other hand, evening primrose oil seems to have few side effects, so it may be worth a try.

Vitamin E was advocated in the past, but is now known *vitamin E is ineffective for breast pain* or lumpiness. Two randomized trials in which women took either vitamin E or placebo (a sugar pill) found no benefit for the women who took vita-min E ####. Earlier experience claiming a benefit had failed to account for the fact that even significant breast pain usually becomes less severe after several months. They had attributed this typical regression of breast pain to the vitamin E, when in fact it is what usually happens with breast pain.

Elimination of caffeine may help reduce breast pain in some women, but there are so many women who drink beverages with caffeine every day and have no sig-nificant breast pain that it is difficult to think of caffeine as a major cause of breast disease. The research trials have shown only minimal or no benefits from reducing coffee intake ####. If you drink many beverages with caffeine and have a lot of breast pain, it may be worth a try, since giving up caffeine is certainly not harmful. It just may not work to alleviate your breast pain.

The real risk in giving up caffeine, taking vitamin E, or taking evening primrose oil is that such simple measures may trivialize the importance of your breast symp-toms. It is OK to try these remedies, but do not let reliance on them take the place of careful evaluation by your physician. If you have new symptoms and your physi-cian cannot find a specific cause, repeat evaluation over time is still a necessary part of being certain that you are healthy.

Remember that most breast pain will get better. The important thing is to be certain that you have a careful breast evaluation if you have new symptoms.

"Will a mammogram help diagnose my pain?"

A mammogram can sometimes show an abnormality that cannot be felt, and such findings may explain pain. It is unwise, however, to say that findings on a mammogram are fibrocystic and rely on this "diagnosis" as the cause of pain.

Because mammograms are not able to detect at least 15% of breast cancers, or a higher percentage if only invasive cancers are counted, a negative mammogram is never completely reliable.

It is best to consider a mammogram as a useful test only if it is positive, and not as part of your decision process if it is negative.

Biopsies

"Do I need a biopsy?"

If there is an area of your breast that is different from the rest of your breast, either on the mammogram, ultrasound, or MRI or on physical examination, you should insist that your physician determine why this is the case. The most reliable way to determine what is happening in an area of your breast is to have a sample taken from that tissue and evaluated by a pathologist who is trained to recognize the signs of cancer under a microscope. This requires a biopsy.

"What kinds of biopsies are there?"

There are four types of biopsies. Three use a needle and one uses surgery with a small scalpel to cut your skin. Each kind of biopsy can be done either with or without the guidance of an imaging technique such as a mammogram, ultrasound, MRI, or a special computer-guided stereotactic biopsy-guiding machine.

1. In a cyst aspiration, a standard size needle (like would be used for a flu shot) is placed into a cyst or fluid-filled mass to remove the fluid. Nothing remains after a cyst aspiration, and if anything remains, another kind of biopsy is necessary.
2. In a fine needle aspiration, a standard size needle is used to remove individual cells from within a solid mass that is not filled with fluid.
3. In a core biopsy, a larger needle is used to remove a small core (about the diameter of a pen refill) of intact tissue.
4. In a surgical biopsy, a small knife, or scalpel, is used to cut the skin, and a surgeon removes a piece of breast tissue for testing.

"Can I have a cyst aspiration?"

Needle aspiration of a cyst is very different from fine needle aspiration and is used for only one, very select, but also relatively common situation. It is used only when there is a suspected cyst that can be felt by hand or seen on an ultrasound. The needle is placed in the cyst and the fluid is removed. Once the fluid is removed, the cyst collapses and there is no mass left. If there is *any mass left after aspiration,* then either a fine needle aspiration or other type of biopsy must be done. If your physician says that he or she is going to aspirate a cyst and no fluid is removed, some other type of biopsy is necessary.

"Can I have a fine needle aspiration biopsy for my lump?"

A fine needle biopsy can determine the nature of a palpable finding. For a needle biopsy to work there must be a specific area to be sampled, and there must be enough material obtained for analysis to be done.

Fine needle aspiration (FNA) uses a small needle to scrape cells loose from inside a lump or area of your breast. These cells are collected in the needle and kept there using gentle suction or aspiration with a syringe. You can think of this as being like a Pap smear of tissue from inside your breast. In fact, the cells are processed and evaluated like a Pap smear. The disadvantage of this technique is that it leaves the lump in place. The advantage is that it samples a larger area than core biopsy and is less painful. The limitation of fine needle aspiration is that to be reliable, a person with special experience must do it.

To interpret an FNA, the pathologist looks at the cytology or the structure of individual cells. If a lump is cancer, the cells from that lump will be cancer. If a lump is not cancer, the cells from that lump will not be cancer. Cells from cancer and cells from benign lumps usually look very different (page 64).

"How much can I rely on a negative fine needle aspiration?"

FNA is usually interpreted as one part of a three-part test called the *triple test*. The triple test consists of physical examination, mammograms, and the fine needle aspiration. If all three indicate that the area is benign, there is greater than 99% accuracy that the area is not cancer ###. If the triple test is negative (not cancer), the fourth part of evaluating a breast abnormality with FNA is to reexamine the area in six months to be certain it has not changed.

"Who is qualified to do a fine needle aspiration?"

In 1996, the National Cancer Institute convened a consensus panel to discuss fine needle aspiration biopsy. The panel heard evidence that FNA is a reliable method to diagnose palpable lumps, i.e., lumps that can be felt. The panel also heard evidence that FNA is most reliable when the FNA biopsy is performed by people who have had special training.

A good index of the ability of a person to do FNA is the rate or percentage of

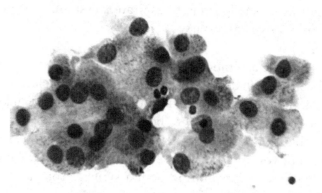

Benign (non- cancerous) breast cells from a fine needle aspiration biopsy. The nucleus of each cell (dark grey) is either round or oval and the nuclei are all about the same size. The nuclei are smaller than the cytoplasm (light grey) of each cell. These are mostly normal luminal cells.

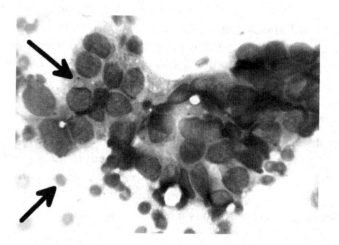

Malignant or cancerous cells from a fine needle aspiration biopsy. The nuclei (dark grey) are much larger and they fill the cells so much that there is only a little cytoplasm (light grey). The nuclei are of different sizes and different shapes and they clump together. Comparison to normal red blood cells (arrows) shows the cancer nuclei are much larger.
Photos courtesy of D. John Abele

their cases that do not have adequate specimens. It is not possible to obtain an adequate specimen of cells from all breast lumps. However, if more than 10% of a physician's FNAs are inadequate, that physician is probably not performing a reliable test. Although it was carefully discussed, this important quality assurance information was not included in the final recommendations of the panel.

"Can I have a core biopsy of my breast?"

Large needle or core biopsy is another way to sample a solid lump. The pathologist studies a broader section of tissue to look both at individual cells (cytology) and the patterns of how the individual cells relate to one another (histology). The disadvantage of this type of biopsy is that it looks at tissue only from a small area so multiple core samples must be taken to avoid missing cancer. The advantage is that most pathologists can interpret the histology of an area tissue whereas special training is required to interpret cytology of individual cells.

"Is my needle or core biopsy concordant with the images?"

If a mammogram, ultrasound, or MRI was used to guide a biopsy, after the pathologist has determined the kind of tissue in the biopsy, the diagnosis, the radiologist will review the results of the pathology report and compare them to the mammogram. If the results of the biopsy are the kind of results that were expected, the biopsy is said to be *concordant*.

If the radiologist was concerned about cancer—for example, it was a Bi-Rads 4 image—and the pathology report is benign, then the results are *not concordant*. Not concordant means that the biopsy needle might have missed a cancer, and usually a surgical biopsy should be done.

"Do I need a surgical biopsy?"

A surgical or open biopsy is usually required if there is any question after a needle biopsy or cyst aspiration. Also, if the needle biopsy is negative (benign), but there is only a minimal sample of tissue or the radiologist or your physician does not have confidence in the negative biopsy, i.e., it is not concordant, an open biopsy is almost always required.

If you have a lump or an unusual area in your breast, but a negative mammogram and physical examination, you should still ask your physician directly if there is any lingering question of whether cancer might be present.

Even a surgical biopsy is not foolproof ###. About one-half of a percent of surgical biopsies will miss a cancer that is in the area. This does not necessarily mean that the wrong *lump* was biopsied. It means that sometimes a cancer can be developing in an area and may not be found by a biopsy. It is important that biopsies be done for specific lesions. Then at least the surgeon can know that the specific area is what is removed. This is the reason that it is not useful to demand a biopsy if there is not a specific area on which your physician can focus or concentrate attention.

If you are worried, but your physician cannot feel a specific area to biopsy, seek another opinion. You can also ask your physician to reexamine you in 8 to12 weeks.

"What if there is a suspicious area on my mammogram and no one can feel it?"

If a suspicious area on a mammogram, MRI, or ultrasound cannot be felt, it is localized with a wire before surgery. Because the radiologist can see the suspicious area on the mammogram - and at the same time see the wire - she or he can position the wire at the area of concern. Your surgeon follows the wire to the area marked by the radiologist. This is called a wire or needle localization.

"If I have had a biopsy that is not cancer, am I now more likely to get cancer in the future?"

A biopsy itself does not increase the risk of cancer, but being in the group of women who have had any kind of surgical breast biopsy is statistically associated with some increase in breast cancer in the future. The kind of tissue found in the biopsy strongly influences future risks. Biopsy tissue that is not cancer can be classified into three groups: nonproliferative, proliferative without atypia, and proliferative with atypia. Both the BCSC and the Gail risk calculators consider whether a biopsy falls into one of these three groups (see page 43).

About 85% of benign breast biopsies are of nonproliferative tissue. If you have a breast biopsy that finds nonproliferative changes, as far as this biopsy can indicate, you do not have an increased risk of getting breast cancer. Stated another way, your risk of getting breast cancer is very similar to that of any other woman of your age.

About 10% of breast biopsies will find proliferative changes without atypia. If this is what your biopsy found, you have a slight increase in the risk of getting breast cancer for the next 15 to 20 years. The relative risk is about 1.2 so if you are, for example, 40 years old, your risk is 1.5% multiplied by 1.2 or about 1.8% instead of 1.5%. Different, but not very different.

About 5% of benign breast biopsies find *atypical hyperplasia or atypical proliferative changes*. If you have had atypical hyperplasia found on a breast biopsy, you have an increased risk of getting breast cancer. In absolute terms, about 15% of women with atypical hyperplasia on a breast biopsy will develop breast cancer within 20 years. (See discussion of relative risk on page 40). Also, if the atypia is on the limited sample from an FNA or a core biopsy, between 25 and 30% of the time cancer will be found in the area if a surgical biopsy is done. Thus, if atypia is found on a core biopsy, a surgical biopsy is recommended to study the area more thoroughly.

Some experts recommend drugs to reduce cancer risk for women with atypia on a biopsy (page 46). There are risks of the treatment itself. However, there are also risks of treatment too late, if cancer develops and it is not recognized early. In general, however, I would consider drugs to prevent cancer only for atypical lesions.

"What is a fibroadenoma?"

A fibroadenoma is a benign tumor that typically occurs in young women although it can occur after menopause. It usually feels very smooth and easily "slips" around in breast tissue. As with any lump, a biopsy should be done to confirm it is benign. It should be removed if it is over 3/4 inches in size or if it regrows.

"If you think the area in my breast is OK, how can you be certain?"

The difficult issue is that even observation over time does not guarantee that cancer is not present or will not develop. Your physician is always trying to balance two issues. The first is to recognize and biopsy an early cancer based on very subtle findings. The second is doing a biopsy of the wrong area or missing a cancer on a biopsy, being misled by a benign biopsy, or worse, having subtle changes or early cancer obscured by a postoperative scar in an area where a biopsy has just been done.

In general, the question that must always be answered is whether your physician can identify a specific area that is different from the rest of your breast. If an area is identified as different, then some sort of sampling of that area should usually be done.

"What should I do next?"

First, ask yourself if you feel satisfied either that the area in question no longer exists or has been sufficiently sampled.

If the answer to either of these questions is "No," then you must ask, "What is the plan?" Repeat observation is always an option, but if this option is chosen, it should be with your agreement.

If you disagree with the recommendation of your physician, or if you just want to feel reassured, it is quite reasonable to ask for a second opinion or a consultation with another physician who will evaluate your breasts from a fresh perspective.

If you ask for another opinion, you will learn a lot about your own physician. A wise physician has come to terms with the fact that she or he is not right every time. In general terms, a physician who will cooperate (or direct their staff to cooperate) with you is a safer physician. A physician who acknowledges individual fallibility is more likely to remain vigilant on your behalf. She or he will know that a second opinion is not a statement that you do not trust your physician. It is a statement that you are realistic and that you need to be vigilant on your own behalf.

PART THREE

QUESTIONS TO ASK IF YOU HAVE BEEN DIAGNOSED WITH BREAST CANCER

Being diagnosed with breast cancer is invariably an intense emotional experience. Virtually everyone diagnosed with breast cancer has powerful feelings that range from fear to anger, or from depression to guilt. The first step to healing is to acknowledge these feelings, and to find ways to begin to move through your emotional response, to deciding what you will choose to do. Information can help you move beyond your fear to taking steps that care for yourself, and seeking information can *begin even in the midst of intense emotions.*

No one can say what will happen to you as an individual. Your physician will be able to tell you whether your cancer has a higher or lower risk of threatening your health, but she or he will not be able to predict the future. People with very bad cancers do survive. Even bad cancers are not always fatal.

Likewise, only you experience your cancer. Your feelings, good or bad, are valid and it is important to be true to your own feelings. Sometimes well-meaning friends will urge you "be positive" but in general you will do best if you acknowledge your own feelings. *There is little value in attempting to force your mind to act one way when it feels another.* It is better to acknowledge the truth of how you feel. It can be therapeutic to scream how unfair it is.

"What are the ways cancer can be dangerous?"
Breast cancer can be dangerous in two ways:

1. Breast cancer can regrow in the breast—or in the area of the breast even after the breast has been removed. This is called a *local recurrence*. Local recurrence can be very unpleasant, but it is rarely fatal by itself.

2. Breast cancer can leave the area of the breast and grow in another part of the body. This growth in another part of the body is called a *metastasis*. A breast cancer metastasis is a great threat to life.

When a physician talks about danger or risks associated with a given cancer, he or she means either the risk of local recurrence, or the risk of metastasis or growth elsewhere in the body, or more commonly, both.

"What kind of cancer do I have?"

There are five kinds of breast cancer. Many other words are used and there are additional descriptions that can be given to cancers within each type, but in terms of what might make a difference to you, almost all breast cancers fall into one of five categories. There are two types of *in situ* cancers (*in situ* is a Latin medical phrase meaning *in the place*) and three types of invasive cancers. Each has its own meaning and implications.

In situ cancers have not yet developed the ability to invade tissue. They cannot make their own space. However, *in situ* cancers can grow in any preexisting space. The ducts of the breast, the tubes that carry milk in a nursing mother, extend through much of the breast and constitute a large preexisting space that extends throughout the same area. In some instances, *in situ* cancer can grow extensively inside these ducts but still cannot break out of the ducts. Because they cannot make their own space, there is minimal risk that *in situ* cancers will spread to another part of a woman's body.

Invasive cancers have developed the ability to break through the wall (or basement membrane) of milk ducts in the breast where virtually all breast cancers start. They can make their own space and grow in other parts of the body. They pose a greater threat to a woman's long-term health.

"What is lobular carcinoma *in situ*?"

Lobular carcinoma *in situ* (also called LCIS or lobular neoplasia) is a noninvasive cancer. Many experts feel that this may not be a real cancer in the sense that it cannot invade normal tissue and it does not metastasize.

No one dies of LCIS unless she develops another, more dangerous invasive cancer. If we start with a group of 100 women with LCIS, about 15 women out of the group will develop invasive cancer over 20 years.

MAGNIFIED VIEW ILLUSTRATING PROGRESSION
FROM NORMAL DUCTS TO INVASIVE CANCER

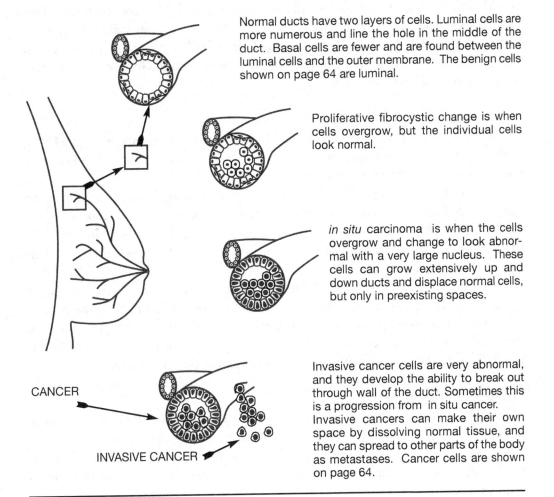

Normal ducts have two layers of cells. Luminal cells are more numerous and line the hole in the middle of the duct. Basal cells are fewer and are found between the luminal cells and the outer membrane. The benign cells shown on page 64 are luminal.

Proliferative fibrocystic change is when cells overgrow, but the individual cells look normal.

in situ carcinoma is when the cells overgrow and change to look abnormal with a very large nucleus. These cells can grow extensively up and down ducts and displace normal cells, but only in preexisting spaces.

CANCER

Invasive cancer cells are very abnormal, and they develop the ability to break out through wall of the duct. Sometimes this is a progression from in situ cancer.
Invasive cancers can make their own space by dissolving normal tissue, and they can spread to other parts of the body as metastases. Cancer cells are shown on page 64.

INVASIVE CANCER

A little more than half of the invasive cancers developing after LCIS will be in the breast where the LCIS was found, and a little less than half develop in the opposite breast. Treatment of the breast where the LCIS was found would leave the other breast (where almost half of the invasive cancers will develop) untreated. For this reason, most experts consider LCIS a marker for a higher risk and design a plan to recheck both breasts on a frequent basis, typically every 6 months.

Neither surgery nor radiation therapy is usually recommended for LCIS. Since cancer in the future can occur in any part of either breast, surgery or radiation would logically require treatment of both breasts since both have equal risk. This would be extreme. Some experts advocate tamoxifen or an aromatase inhibitor for LCIS, but this must be considered in the context of other health issues. A woman with LCIS should have a careful plan for follow-up as outlined for high-risk women in Parts One and Two of this book.

"What is ductal carcinoma *in situ?*"

Ductal carcinoma *in situ* (also called DCIS or intraductal cancer) is like LCIS, in that in its pure form it does not have the ability to invade tissue. However, *it is more dangerous right where it is found.*

It is more common for DCIS to be mixed with very small amounts of invasive cancer, called micro-invasion. When these areas of micro-invasion occur, it means that the cancer has begun to invade normal tissue and there is a small but real risk of metastases. Even in the absence of micro-invasion, DCIS seems to be more dangerous than LCIS.

If we start with a group of 100 women with DCIS, within 20 years about 15 will have developed an invasive breast cancer. However, unlike LCIS, most cancers will have developed *in the same area* as the original DCIS. Because DCIS is linked to a risk of invasive cancer in the area of the breast where the DCIS started, it is generally agreed that this part of a woman's breast should be treated.

"How is DCIS treated?"

DCIS is usually removed from the breast surgically. For small DCIS this is done with a wide local excision like for invasive cancer (see page 84). For large DCIS, a mastectomy may be the better choice. There is some experimentation with trying to shrink DCIS with drugs before surgery, but this is not an established treatment at this time.

"Is ductal carcinoma *in situ* pre-cancer or early cancer?"

The word *cancer* has an implied social and emotional meaning that is surprisingly uniform across cultures and languages. It denotes a disease which, untreated, threatens life with pain and visible destruction of body tissues. In its advanced stages, breast cancer is visible as it draws in and destroys surrounding tissue. This destruction of normal tissue reminded our ancestors of a crab or another claw-bearing crustacean, so they named *cancer* using their words for such crustaceans, most often a crab ("cancer" is Latin for "crab"). When a physician says "cancer", she or he taps into this deeply ingrained social and emotional meaning.

Ductal carcinoma *in situ* is an early step in a continuum of changes in breast tissue that can eventually become a disease that has all of the tissue-damaging properties associated with cancer. It is not the first step and it is unclear whether it is always an early step in this progression to cancer.

In the sense that, without treatment, DCIS can progress to a disease that threatens life with the possibility of pain and destruction of tissues, DCIS is early cancer. However, not all DCIS will progress to such a destructive cancer.

Given the fact that not all DCIS will progress to a destructive cancer, some experts insist that it is only pre-cancer. Other experts, however, say that this inappropriately understates the risks of DCIS and insist that DCIS should be called early cancer.

A recent study looked at the long-term results after treatment of DCIS in the national SEER database (SEER is explained in the glossary). After 20 years, 3% of women with DCIS died from breast cancer which is much lower mortality than for any other breast cancer. Some commentators argue that this proves that DCIS is pre cancer because there is such excellent prognosis, but that is not logical because over 95% of women in the study had been treated to eliminate the original DCIS.

If you have DCIS, the important consideration is to understand the possibility that it might progress to cancer that threatens your life. If there is only DCIS and no invasive cancer, lymph nodes are not usually removed and chemotherapy is not used. Hormone therapy is often recommended if the DCIS has hormone receptors (see page 79). The exception is if a mastectomy is done for extensive DCIS, a sentinel node (see page 89) is usually removed.

"How dangerous is my DCIS?"

Ductal carcinoma *in situ* can be graded using various systems. A similar system called the Scarf-Bloom-Richardson grading system is used for invasive cancers. (See page 77).

One system developed by Silverstein and Lagios, the Van Nuys Scale, estimates the risk that the DCIS will re-grow in your breast. It was originally based on three elements:

- The size of the DCIS.
- The distance between the cancer cells and the edge of the tissue removed (the size of the margins).
- The visible nature of the pathology of the cancer cells, which is called grade and is similar to the degree of variability of cells in the Scarf-Bloom-Richardson scale for invasive cancers (*see page 77*).

There are other systems to score DCIS and there is not consensus that the Van Nuys scale is the best. However, the Van Nuys scale is simple, and seems to be reproducible between different hospitals.

For the Van Nuys scale, a score of 1 to 3 is assigned for each aspect of the cancer as follows:

Size of the DCIS

Less than or equal to 1.5 cm	1 point
1.6 to 4.0 cm	2 points
4.1 cm or larger	3 points

Margins of the DCIS excision

More than 1.0 cm	1 point
0.1 to 0.9 cm	2 points
Less than 0.1 cm	3 points

Visible cancer pathology

Non–high-grade, without dead cells	1 point
Non–high-grade, with dead cells	2 points
High-grade	3 points

(For invasive cancers, see page 77, "What grade is my cancer?")

A score of 1 to 3 is assigned for each characteristic. These scores added together give a total from 3 to 9. Tumors with a score of 3 or 4 are unlikely to grow back in the breast. Tumors with a score of 5, 6, or 7 will usually not re grow if radiation therapy is given. Tumors with a score of 8 or 9 often re grow unless the entire breast is removed.

A newer version of the Van Nuys scale includes age over or under 50 years. Women over 50 have more risk of local recurrence.

An important aspect of this scoring system for DCIS is that the size of the margins can be changed with further surgery. For example, a tumor with a margin of less than 0.1 cm (3 points for margins) and a total score of 8 can be converted to a score of 6 if more surgery is done and a margin of 1.0 cm of tissue is removed (only 1 point for margins). The question to consider before attempting more surgery is how much breast tissue will have been removed after another operation, and then, what will the remaining breast look like?

There is also much current opinion that the size of margins does not matter if radiation therapy is given to the remainder of the breast. It must be emphasized, however, that narrow margins can only be accepted if radiation therapy is part of the treatment plan.

"What are the types of invasive cancer?"

• Invasive ductal cancer is the most common type of breast cancer. It is dangerous and presents a real risk of metastasis. It usually grows in only one part of a woman's breast, but invasive ductal cancer can occur in more than one part of a woman's breast and it can occur in the opposite breast. When it is small and only in one part of a woman's breast, it can be treated without removing the breast. Invasive ductal cancers come in almost as many types as there are patients. In general, it is best to try to understand whether the cancer has or does not have any particularly dangerous characteristics. There are several subtypes of invasive ductal cancer. Some specialized types have a very good prognosis. Invasive ductal cancers are often grouped as Luminal A, Luminal B, HER2 type, and triple negative (see page 80).

• Invasive lobular cancer differs from invasive ductal cancer mainly in how it spreads through the breast. Invasive lobular cancer lacks a protein called E-Cadherin that tends to hold cells together and thus it is more likely to spread widely in little bits of tumor throughout the breast. The tendency to spread as little bits or rows of cancer cells makes it more difficult to detect by examination or mammogram and may make larger invasive lobular cancers difficult to remove and still leave any breast tissue behind. Invasive lobular cancer is slightly more likely to appear in the other breast than invasive ductal cancer. Otherwise, it is very similar to invasive ductal cancer.

•Inflammatory breast cancer is the third type of invasive cancer. Technically it is a type of invasive ductal or lobular cancer, but its diagnosis and clinical behavior are distinctly different so inflammatory breast cancer is usually considered by itself. It is relatively uncommon, but it is extremely dangerous and spreads rapidly. Inflammatory cancer makes the breast red and it is often mistaken for an infection in its early phases. If you have been diagnosed as having inflammatory cancer (usually by a skin biopsy that shows cancer cells in the skin itself), your physician will assume that you have early metastases, even if tests are negative. She or he will usually recommend that you have treatment for your whole body (chemotherapy) before trying to treat the cancer area in the breast itself.

"Where is my cancer located at this time?"

The specific location of a cancer *in the breast* has little significance in how dangerous a cancer is, except that tumors near the sternum or breastbone can sometimes metastasize to lymph nodes inside the chest. This location is hard to detect. What makes a difference is the size of the cancer and where, if anywhere, it has spread out of the breast.

Cancer can be located in more than one part of the breast. This is called multifocal or multicentric. Multicentric cancers are more likely to have local recurrence, but they are not more likely to have a metastasis unless one of the single parts is also bigger.

Cancer can spread (metastasize) to areas outside the breast. The most easily identified metastases are found in lymph nodes near the breast, either in the axilla (armpit) or, rarely, inside the chest. If cancer is located in any place other than where it started in the breast or the breast ducts, it is a metastasis. Once a cancer has any metastasis, it is more dangerous.

In more advanced cases, cancer can be located in parts of the body away from the breast. For small cancers in the breast, it is uncommon to find spread of cancer to other parts of your body. However your physician should do some simple tests such as a chest X-ray and blood tests of liver function anyway. Areas at higher risk for breast cancer metastases are lungs, bones, liver, and brain.

The *stage* of a cancer summarizes all the places where it is located at that time. Stage I is a smaller cancer that is only in the local area of the breast. Stage II is a little larger and/ or with spread to a few nodes. Stage III is larger and/ or with spread to a lot of nodes, but the cancer is still only in the breast area. Stage IV is a larger cancer that has spread to parts of the body beyond the breast and/ or the local lymph nodes

Describing Breast Cancer for Personalized Medicine

Cancers are described several different ways: by size, grade, proliferation rate, tumor markers, tumor types, and tumor prognostic scores.

"How big is my cancer?"

Size is closely linked with the outcome of invasive breast cancers. Invasive breast cancers are described in three sizes.

- T1 is up to 2 cm in diameter.
- T2 is from 2 cm to 5 cm.
- T3 is larger than 5 cm.
- T4 is any size with extension to the skin or invasion into the chest wall. Officially, inflammatory breast cancer is T4, but it is sufficiently aggressive that it is usually spoken of as a separate entity.

Larger size means two things. First, it is more likely that the cancer will have a local recurrence. It is also more likely that the cancer has been present for a long enough time for some cancer cells to have left the breast and begun to grow as a metastasis elsewhere in a woman's body.

For *in situ* cancers, particularly DCIS, larger size means that more tissue must be removed to remove the cancer. But, since the cancer is not yet invasive, larger size does not always mean a greater chance that an *in situ* cancer has begun to metastasize, or spread elsewhere in the body.

"What grade is my cancer?"

Physicians use the Scarf-Bloom-Richardson grade to describe how a cancer looks under a microscope. The pathologist looks for three characteristics of the cancer and assigns a score of 1, 2, or 3 for each characteristic. The numbers for each of these are added together. The total cannot be less than 3 nor can it be more than 9. The three characteristics used for the scale are:

- Tubule formation
- Mitoses
- Cellular differentiation

Normal breasts make *tubules,* or small tubes, that carry milk. If a cancer still makes tubules, it has not deviated too far from normal and receives a score of 1. If there are no tubules, it has deviated a lot and receives a score of 3 for tubule formation.

For cancer to grow, individual cells grow and then divide into new cells. The process of one cell dividing into two cells is called *mitosis.* Normal breast tissue does not have many dividing or mitotic cells. If there are few mitoses, then the cancer is close to normal and receives a score of 1. If there are a lot of mitoses, the cancer is further from normal and receives a score of 3.

Normal cells have a very typical appearance and look very much the same. If cancer cells are very similar, then they receive a score of 1. If the cells have many different shapes they are called *pleomorphic* and they receive a score of 3. Very pleomorphic cells are illustrated in the picture of an FNA from cancer (page 64). If the cancer has intermediate tubule formation, mitoses, or cell differentiation, it receives a score of 2 for that characteristic.

The numbers for the three characteristics are added and the number used to assign a grade. For example, a tumor might have a lot of tubules (score 1), few mitoses (score 1), and fairly similar cells (score 1), for a total score of 3, which is a grade I cancer. At the other extreme, a cancer might have no tubules (score 3), many mitoses (score 3), and very bizarrely shaped cells (score 3), for a total of 9 points, which is a grade III cancer.

Grade I tumor	Total of 3 to 5 points	Most favorable
Grade II tumor	Total of 6 to 7 points	Intermediate
Grade III tumor	Total of 8 or 9 points	Least favorable

A grade III cancer is dangerous even if it is both T1 and has no node involvement. The high Scarf-Bloom-Richardson grade indicates a danger of metastasis even if the cancer is otherwise small. However, a high tumor grade is not a reason to do a mastectomy to reduce chances of local recurrence. Grade has little influence on local recurrence once the cancer is fully removed. (See page 83).

"Does my cancer have hormone receptors?"

Hormone receptors (estrogen receptors or ERs and progesterone receptors or PRs) have been measured for invasive breast cancers for years (more recently they are also measured on DCIS). These tests tell whether the individual cells of a cancer still behave like normal breast duct cells in that they grow if they are given estrogen and slow or stop growth if estrogens are blocked or taken away. Presence of ER and PR is also a favorable prognostic sign.

If a tumor has estrogen receptors it is said to be *ER positive*, and similarly for a *PR positive* cancer.

If any hormone receptors are present the tumor is called *hormone receptor* positive and hormone-based treatments are recommended. However, if the tumor is only weakly positive it is not as good a sign as if the tumor is strongly positive. Similarly, a tumor that is ER positive but PR negative is more dangerous than one that is both ER and PR positive

"How fast is my cancer growing?"

Cancer grows only when individual cells within the tumor divide, and the growth rate tells how fast a cancer will progress. Growth rate is typically reported as the percentage of cells in the *growth fraction*. The growth fraction is identified because the cells contain a protein called Ki-67. (Ki-67 is identified with antibodies such as MIB1, and some laboratories report Ki-67 as the percent of cells that react with MIB1.) An average growth fraction is about 20 to 25%. Higher growth fraction means the cancer is more dangerous.

Growth can also be identified by measuring the cells that are *synthesizing* new DNA to prepare to divide. These cells are said to be in *S-phase* (S for synthesis). Like the growth fraction, the percent of cells in S-phase tells if the cancer is fast-growing.

"Does my cancer over-express HER2?"

HER2 is a gene that makes protein on the surface of cancer cells. This protein (p185) receives a signal for the cell to grow when the cell is exposed to growth factors. Growth factors are small proteins released into tissue to signal other cells to grow; growth factors are always present in some amount in most tissues. Therefore when the protein p185 on a cancer cell is exposed to growth factors, it tells the cancer to grow.

Between 20 and 30% of breast cancers have cells with increased amounts of HER2 because the gene that directs the cell to make HER2 has increased in number. This is called *over-expression* of the HER2 gene. These cells are more responsive to growth factors and, therefore, these cancers are more aggressive. Women with cancers that over-express HER2 are more likely to develop metastases. The prognosis, based on these studies, is more serious and additional therapy is beneficial.

Pathologists test for HER2 in two steps: First, very thin tissue slices are stained with antibodies that make the HER2 protein look different. If the HER2 protein is either clearly present (said to be positive) or clearly absent, other testing can be omitted. If the results are not clearly positive or negative, a different test is done to evaluate the exact number of copies of the HER2 gene.

The drugs trastuzumab (brand name Herceptin) and pertuzumab (brand name Perjeta) can neutralize the negative effects of over-expression of HER2.

"What molecular subtype of tumor do I have?"

Ductal cancers are often classified using a combination of the individual scores for estrogen receptors, progesterone receptors, and HER2. The basis for these cancer types is that benign breast cells grow in two layers (page 71), cells close to the lumen or hole in the middle of the ducts—called luminal—and cells away from the lumen, around the wall of the ducts, that are called basal. Cancers that arise or come from the basal cells are more dangerous.

The cells from which a cancer originated can be guessed by the combination of the ER, PR, and HER2 tests. The results are not precise, but these markers provide good estimates of treatment benefits and risks of recurrence.

Markers are combined in order of increasing risk as follows:

Luminal A - the most favorable type, is ER positive, PR positive, and HER2 negative.

Luminal B - Less favorable variant of hormone receptor positive that can happen two ways: either ER positive, PR positive, and HER2 positive, or ER positive, PR positive, and high growth fraction (high Ki-67).

HER2 type - ER negative, PR negative, and HER2 positive.

Basal type - also called "triple negative" is the most dangerous type. It is ER negative, PR negative, and HER2 negative.

"What is my prognostic score?"

There are several commercial prognostic-scoring systems that measure the expression or activity of several genes in a sample of the cancer tissue, and use the combined results to estimate the risk that the cancer will metastasize. These scores are often used to predict possible benefits of chemotherapy when a woman has no cancer in her lymph nodes and the tumor is ER positive or larger size.

The first system is the 21-gene assay. It is often used to estimate risks of recurrence if only hormone treatments are given for a hormone responsive (ER+ and/ or PR+) cancer, and is reported as a score from 1 to 50. The score is used to predict the benefit of adding chemotherapy to hormone treatment. For a 21-gene score of 10 or less, the risk is low and chemotherapy can usually be omitted.

The 70-gene assay (similar in concept to the 21-gene score but marketed by another company) works on the same principle, but provides a single score that recommends either for or against adding chemotherapy to other treatment. As for the 21-gene assay, a low 70-gene assay indicates that chemotherapy adds minimal benefit and can usually be omitted.

General Principles for Treatment of Breast Cancer.

Two basic principles that guide all recommendations for breast cancer:
1. What do we know from past experience about the risks that this patient faces?
2. What benefit can we reasonably anticipate from each kind of therapy that can be used?

These questions are useful because the benefit from any specific treatment is usually in proportion to the risk that the cancer had at the beginning. For example, preventing half of the spread (metastases) in a patient with a 50% chance of spread will be life-changing for the 25% of women who benefit (half of 50% is 25%). However, if the same therapy is given to women with a 10% chance of spread, only 5% of women will benefit (half of 10% is 5%).

However, it is important to observe that *half is also the same as 50%*. Thus in both of these examples, it would be technically correct to say that the treatment reduced the risk of spread by 50%; but this 50% is only half of whatever the risk was to begin with. This distinction is important because sometimes doctors will say a treatment reduces recurrence by 50%. This might be understood to predict much more benefit than would actually happen.

If you want to know what benefit to expect from any treatment, always *ask what is the absolute benefit* of the treatment. (This is a lot like relative risk and absolute risk when describing risk factors on page 40). Thinking about the example above, the first person with the 50% chance of recurrence (spread) would be 25% more likely to do well in absolute terms, and it's likely that benefit will be worth the challenges of taking the treatment. The second woman, however—the woman who started with a 10% risk—was going to do better in the first place. She would only get an actual benefit of 5% better survival; and she may decide that gain does not outweigh the side effects of treatment.

In surveys, women who've had chemotherapy would usually go through it again for a 5% benefit, but not for less. Some might choose to skip a therapy that has minimal benefit. That is a personal choice. Your physician's role is to explain the absolute risks from the treatment and the absolute benefits expected from the treatment so that you can make your own decision.

"What are the central challenges in treating breast cancer?"

There are two main challenges in treating breast cancer:

1. *Eliminate the source where the cancer started.* The cancer in the breast itself is called the *primary tumor* because is the first location or the source of the cancer. As long as cancer exists in the breast, cells can separate from the cancer and travel or spread though blood or lymph vessels to other parts of the body.

The breast is usually treated with a combination of surgery, radiation therapy, and/or hormone or chemotherapy. Small cancers are often removed from the breast right away, and the breast itself is preserved. Larger cancers can be treated by removing the breast (mastectomy) or by treating the cancer with drugs to make it small enough that it can be removed and the rest of the breast can be left in place. (Giving drugs as the first treatment of a large cancer works because the drugs not only can shrink the primary tumor, but they follow cancer cells into the blood and kill them there, too.)

2. *Prevent or treat any possible metastasis,* i.e., spread or growth of the cancer outside of the breast itself. Using a combination of pathology reports, e.g. from lymph nodes, in combination with results of imaging such as chest X-rays, bone scans, PET Scans, CT scans, etc., physicians look for evidence of any cancer outside

the breast. If there is no evidence of cancer at the time, physicians use the same data to estimate the possibility that cancer—cancer that is not evident now—will grow in another part of the body in the future.

"Do I need tests before surgery or other treatments?"

Metastases are more dangerous to a woman's life than the amount of cancer in the breast. If metastases are present, most physicians treat them before doing any surgery on your breast except for a biopsy or removal of just the lump. Fortunately, it is uncommon to find metastases when small cancers are diagnosed; but a brief standard check is almost always indicated or appropriate. Usually it is sufficient to do a chest X-ray and a few blood tests to evaluate liver function and look for signs of bone damage.

Tests such as bone scans and computerized axial tomograms (CAT) studies of the chest or liver are positive in only very few women with early breast cancer (less than 5%). Most experts feel that these tests are inappropriate for small tumors if a woman has a negative chest X-ray and normal liver function tests.

If the chest X-ray or blood tests are positive, bone scans, CAT scans, PET/ CT scans, MRI of the brain, etc. may be appropriate. Scans may also be appropriate before treatment when the tumor is large, there are large axillary nodes, or if a woman has new symptoms such as bone pain, cough, headaches, etc. These signs are uncommon.

Surgery

"Do I need surgery?"

If detectable cancer is not removed from the breast area, it will often grow. Untreated cancer can eventually make an ulcer in the skin and become very uncomfortable. Trials were run in the 1960s treating breast cancer with radiation therapy alone. About half of the cancers would shrink with radiation alone, but the majority of those that shrunk would regrow within 6 to 18 months. Usually it is wiser to remove at least the detectable cancer from the breast.

Sometimes your physician will suspect there is residual cancer in your breast after the mass of a cancer has been removed. If these areas are so very small that they cannot be found with a microscope, they are usually successfully treated with radiation therapy.

"If I choose surgery, how much tissue should be removed from my breast?"

Remove whatever is necessary to remove the cancer from the breast. For large cancers this may be a mastectomy. For small cancers it is usually possible to remove only the cancer and surrounding tissue. If guidelines for margins and radiation therapy are followed, the success of removing the cancer only is usually as good as for doing an entire mastectomy.

Comparison of Success of Early Breast Cancer Treatment

Relative Amount of Tissue Removed	Treatment	Success Rate
	Remove lump only (cancer-positive margin)	50%
	Remove lump + radiation therapy	80%
	Remove lump with wide margins (free of cancer)	80%
	Remove lump with wide margins + radiation therapy	95%
	Remove entire breast	96%

"How does a surgeon know how much tissue to remove?"

Your surgeon will ask the pathologist to evaluate the margins of the tissue that is removed from your breast to be certain that the margins are negative for the presence of cancer.

"What are margins?"

The margin is the part of the tissue your surgeon removed that's between the cancer and the tissue that is *still inside you*. It is usually measured as the width of tissue between the cancer and the edge of the tissue that was removed.

Cancer tends to spread out in the breast tissue, so that the last cancer cells are usually several millimeters or more from the lump of a cancer itself. These last cancer cells often are in tissue that looks normal. Therefore, at the time of surgery, your surgeon should remove a rim of normal-appearing tissue around the cancer to be certain to have a good chance of obtaining a negative margin.

After cancer is removed, the pathologist puts permanent ink on the surface of the tissue before slides are cut for examination under the microscope. The pathologist looks at the tissue under the microscope and determines how close the cancer cells are to the ink. If there are cancer cells at the ink, the pathologist knows that the cancer was on the surface (at the ink) of the piece of tissue removed by the surgeon. If there are cancer cells on the surface, it is very likely that other cancer cells are still left in the woman's body. This is called a *positive margin*, and more surgery is recommended. If there are no cancer cells near the margin of the original piece of tissue removed, or if a second surgery obtains negative margins, then no further surgery is recommended for the breast.

Women who have their cancer removed with negative margins have the same chance of living after their cancer as women who have their whole breast removed.

Sometimes a physician will argue that a tumor is too large or in a bad place (such as the nipple area) and that a mastectomy with reconstruction will look better. The decision about what will *look better* is all in your personal viewpoint. There is no medical reason to say that you need a mastectomy, except if the amount of tissue that must be removed to obtain negative margins is so big that there is only minimal breast tissue left or that the breast will be greatly deformed. Even this is still a judgment call and you are the judge.

The appropriate question is not *Do I need a mastectomy?* but rather *What will my breast look like after all of the cancer is removed?* Then you can decide what you want.

"How wide must my negative margin be?"

In the past, knowing that only a sample of the margins could ever be evaluated, many surgeons (myself included) advocated a minimum of two millimeters of cancer-free tissue between the last cancer cell and the ink.

A consensus panel has concluded that "no cancer on ink" is a sufficient margin. They recommend accepting the thickness of one cell between the last cancer cell and ink.

It is important to know that a consensus panel is a group of doctors who sit in a room and create a recommendation based on their collective *opinion*. It is an opinion based on reading a lot of studies, but it is still an opinion. For margins, it is an opinion that has been widely accepted, but this is not a simple issue.

"Why would a consensus panel recommend accepting margins that used to be unacceptable?"

It has been known for a long time that if the pathologist finds a narrow margin with cancer cells close to the edge of the specimen, there will be more local regrowth of cancer.

The panel argues, however, that a narrow margin leads to more regrowth of cancer in the breast *only if no other treatment is given*. Currently almost every patient receives some form of drug as adjuvant therapy (see page 94 for discussion of adjuvant therapy), and adjuvant therapy reduces local recurrence of cancer beyond the reduction from radiation alone after removal of the cancer from the breast. Thus narrower margins will work out okay for patients if they receive adjuvant therapy and radiation therapy.

The panel also argues that insisting on wider margins means that up to 30% of women—depending on how widely the surgeon removes the cancer in the first place—will require further surgery to achieve wider margins, and more surgery adds costs. Striving for wider margins also affects how much tissue is removed. For example, a surgeon has the best chance of a negative margin, free from cancer, when more tissue is removed. However, removing more tissue affects the cosmetic appearance of the breast, which gets worse as more tissue is removed.

"Are there exceptions to the consensus panel recommendations?"

Most breast surgeons in a recent survey accepted the panel's recommendations most of the time. However, surgeons also recognized situations where the panel's opinion is not best for the patient: If a cancer is high grade such as a triple-negative cancer, about half would recommend more surgery if the initial margin was less than 2 mm. If the initial surgery found either a lot of DCIS or a lot of invasive lobular cancer close to, but not at the margin, about half would also recommend more surgery.

I personally agree with those surgeons who accept the general concept from the panel, but whose experience also tells them that *there are exceptions to every rule.*

"Is there a way to make my cancer smaller so I can have less surgery?"

Although it is necessary to remove all the cancer that can be found at surgery, it is quite acceptable to use drugs to shrink a large cancer before removing it. For example, with cancers that are small relative to the size of the patient's breast, it is usually recommended to proceed straight to surgical removal (with exceptions noted under neoadjuvant therapy below). However, if a cancer is so large that removing it would cause major deformity of the remaining breast, it is acceptable to use drugs to shrink the cancer before it is removed ####. This is called *neoadjuvant therapy.*

"If I have neoadjuvant therapy, what will that tell me about my cancer?"

In theory, if treatment with chemotherapy or hormone therapy makes a cancer shrink, that should predict whether cancer cells elsewhere in the body have been reduced in the same way. In medical experience, however, it has been difficult to prove that results of neoadjuvant therapy predict what a woman can expect for her cancer.

Recent evidence suggests that how a cancer responds to neoadjuvant therapy provides information about how the patient will do in the future. If there is no remaining cancer in the breast after neoadjuvant therapy—called a *pathological complete response* (a path CR or pCR)—there is a one-third smaller chance of recurrence. Pathologic complete response is seen most often with HER2 positive cancers.

Lymph Nodes

"Do I need to have lymph nodes removed?"

The presence or absence of cancer in your lymph nodes is the best guide as to whether your cancer has started to spread; removal of nodes to look for early signs of metastasis is called *staging.* Your physician can make a good guess of whether there is cancer in your nodes by feeling under your arm, but this guess will be only about 70% accurate.

Cancer can spread without being in your nodes, but in most cases what is going on in your nodes is a tiny sample of what is going on in other areas of your body where a metastasis might grow. Your physician cannot remove parts of your lungs or liver to look for metastasis, but he or she can remove some nodes with limited harm to you.

Lymph node removal has very specific complications of arm swelling, limitations of arm movement, numbness under the arm, and/or pain. These side effects occur directly in proportion to the extent of the node tissue removed. The worst side effect is lymphedema, a chronic, often permanent swelling of the arm where the nodes are removed. Minor side effects are arm stiffness, which is usually temporary, and permanent loss of nerve sensation under the arm (which usually does not interfere with a normal life the way lymphedema does). The more nodes removed, the more likely is some arm swelling, or other side effects. These complications occur in more than 10% of women if they have a complete node dissection.

There is a lot of discussion among oncologists about whether all women with breast cancer should have nodes removed. Some cancers have such a low likelihood of being in even one node that it is not even appropriate to do the surgery that would remove the nodes for the pathologist to examine.

Your surgeon should not remove nodes for an LCIS or small DCIS.

Some physicians believe nodes should not be removed for small, favorable invasive cancers either. It is not wrong to suggest leaving nodes for favorable invasive cancers. The problem is that there is no consensus on which favorable cancers might have node dissection omitted.

"What nodes should I have removed?"

How to address nodes depends on whether nodes are palpable or suspicious for metastasis. If there are nodes that feel like they might contain cancer, they should be biopsied or removed. If no suspicious nodes are felt, i.e., the axilla (armpit) is clinically negative, then sentinel node biopsy is used.

"What is a sentinel node biopsy?"

There are many nodes in the axilla of all people. However, only a few of those nodes are connected directly to the breast. The connection is by tiny tubes called *lymphatics* that carry fluid from the breast to the nodes, and these nodes are called *sentinel nodes.* Lymphatics are part of your normal anatomy, so dye or radioactive material will go to the node(s) whether or not cancer has spread to the node. Your doctors want to know if there is cancer in the sentinel nodes because if cancer spreads, it will go first to the sentinel nodes.

The *sentinel node biopsy* uses injection of radioactive material, a blue dye that can be seen, or both, into the breast. The dye or radioactive material goes through the lymphatics to the sentinel node(s), and your surgeon uses a small, surgical incision in the axilla (armpit) to locate the nodes to which the radioactive material or dye has gone.

If the sentinel node is negative (has no cancer), then it is not necessary to remove other nodes.

"What happens if my sentinel node is positive (contains cancer)?"

When sentinel nodes were first used, it was recommended that if the sentinel node contained cancer, a complete axillary dissection should be done since that was considered to be the standard. Since sentinel node biopsy was considered to be an abbreviated form of removing axillary nodes, this is called a *completion axillary lymph node dissection.*

SENTINEL NODE IDENTIFICATION

3. SENTINEL NODE is indicated by the blue dye or radioactive material that came through lymphatics, to the axilla, from the area of the cancer in the breast.

1. INJECTION of blue dye or radioactive material into the breast near the cancer.

2. NORMAL LYMPHATICS carry blue dye or radioactive material to the sentinel node. Note that lymphatics exist in everyone, and passage of dye or isotope through a lymphatic does not indicate spread of cancer.

A randomized controlled trial has now shown that if adjuvant therapy (chemotherapy or hormone therapy or both) *and* radiation therapy are given, there is no benefit of doing a completion axillary dissection ####. So far, this is proven for treatment where only part of the breast is removed and radiation therapy of the remaining breast tissue is a definite part of the treatment plan. This does not apply to mastectomy without radiation therapy.

Other trials are underway to find out if completion axillary dissection can be safely omitted if radiation therapy is not being given. This would be, for example, if a woman has chosen to have a mastectomy instead of breast conserving treatment.

"What are the side effects of removing axillary nodes?"

The most important side effect of removing axillary nodes is lymphedema, a chronic swelling of the arm that must always be managed for the rest of a woman's life. Lesser side effects are tightness or stiffness of the shoulder and/or loss of nerve sensation or numbness under the upper arm.

The extent of side effects of node removal are directly in proportion to the extent of the node tissue removed. However, It is impossible for your surgeon to identify in advance how many nodes she or he will remove or to know the number of nodes removed at the time of surgery unless individual nodes are removed and counted as surgery proceeds. This is because nodes are obscured or buried in fatty tissue, so your surgeon often does not see individual nodes. Usually your surgeon will first define structures such as nerves and blood vessels that should be preserved and then remove the tissue around these structures, knowing that the nodes will be in the tissue that is removed.

Surgeons define three levels of nodes that can be removed:
- Level one is lower and more toward your side.
- Level two is just behind the major muscle at the front of your armpit.
- Level three is very high in your armpit or axilla.

If only level one nodes are removed, there is very low chance of lymphedema. If all three levels are removed, there is up to a 40% risk of arm edema.

Studies have shown that it is unusual (less than 1% of the time) to have a positive node in level three and negative nodes in both level one and two. For this reason, many surgeons do not remove the top level of nodes, ever. The probability of cancer in level two or three with nothing in the lowest level is about 15%. Some surgeons think that this is a low enough possibility that they remove only lower nodes, while some surgeons believe that this leaves too great a risk of missing cancer.

Your input is as valuable as your physician's in deciding whether the extra information from removing more nodes is worth the extra risk of additional surgery.

"Is there a benefit in removing my nodes?"

It is difficult to prove there is benefit, other than information, in removing nodes. One randomized trial assigned women either to have all nodes removed or none removed and found no difference in how long these women lived ####. However, many of the women who were not supposed to have nodes removed had nodes—presumably larger nodes—removed by their surgeon anyway. Thus, this was not a perfect study of whether it is necessary to remove all nodes, and there might be a small benefit to removing at least the bigger nodes (usually in level one) that might contain cancer.

There is also the possibility of a benefit of removing nodes that is unrelated to survival. For example, if cancer grows in a node under the arm, it can be painful or cause arm swelling.

The consensus has been that removal of nodes does not have a therapeutic benefit. However, two studies have demonstrated better survival if local regrowth of cancer was reduced by radiation therapy after a mastectomy ####. One of these studies had only women with positive nodes. The other included women with negative nodes but with tumors larger than five centimeters or ones that had grown into the skin or muscle.

These results suggest that cancer might spread from residual cancer left in a node in the breast area. This explanation is still debated; but if cancer could spread from a lymph node, then there might be a benefit of removing cancer-containing nodes, because surgery is an effective way to eliminate cancer in a node. For this reason, if there is any node that might be involved with cancer based on the way it feels, it is usually removed.

Radiation Therapy

"Why is radiation therapy given after a 'lumpectomy'?"

About 30% of women who have a lumpectomy have another, small, unidentified, cancer somewhere in the breast. Thus, years ago, when surgeons began to do "lumpectomies" the cancers that we could not find were *treated* with radiation therapy. For younger women, for larger cancers, and/or for more aggressive cancer, radiation is almost always the best choice.

"What is partial breast irradiation?"

Local recurrence—regrowth of cancer in the breast after a wide local excision— is uncommon. When it happens, most of the time, cancer regrows in the same area where cancer was first located. Some physicians have suggested that, since cancer rarely regrows in other parts of the breast, radiation is only necessary in the area of the breast where the cancer started. Radiation of only the area where the cancer began—instead of the entire breast—is called *partial breast radiation.*

Partial breast radiation can be given several ways: 1) intraoperatively or during the surgery, 2) after surgery through a special balloon left in the breast at surgery, or 3) by giving a small beam of radiation therapy from many angles so that only the place where the beam focuses receives a therapeutic amount of radiation.

Partial breast radiation therapy is under active investigation. Typically is has been used for less dangerous cancers in older women. Ask your physician for up-to-date information.

"Can some women skip radiation therapy after lumpectomy?"

It turns out that with adjuvant therapy, for a few carefully selected women, these possible, unidentified cancers might not be as important as we thought.

To emphasize, *all women get some benefit from radiation therapy,* but some women do so well that they get *very little benefit from adding radiation therapy.* Generally, these women meet *all* of these criteria: they are over 60 years of age (in some studies over 70), with small (less than one centimeter) well-differentiated, in-filtrating ductal cancers that are strongly ER and PR positive, HER2 negative, have a low growth fraction (Ki-67 under 15%), and have no tumor in axillary nodes.

In an Italian study, the risk of local regrowth in the breast was 3.4% at 9 years with radiation therapy and 4.4 % without radiation therapy. In an English study, the observed recurrence was 3% with radiation therapy and 8% without. In an American study, the 12-year local recurrence was 2% with radiation and 10% with tamoxifen and no radiation. Survival was the same with or without radiation therapy in all three studies, i.e., radiation did not improve survival.

Regarding long-term survival, in the NSABP-06 trial, the biggest trial ever of lumpectomy, half of the women who kept their breast did not receive radiation therapy. Those women definitely had *more local recurrence without radiation,* i.e., regrowth of cancer in the breast, but there was no significant difference in survival for at least the first 18 years.

"Do I need radiation therapy if I have had a mastectomy?"

A complete mastectomy does not guarantee that cancer will not grow back in the area where the breast was located. Even after the most careful surgery, cancer can regrow as a local recurrence on the chest wall up to 3% to 5% of the time. These local recurrences usually grow from tiny bits of residual cancer that are left in the remaining skin after the mastectomy.

Local recurrence after a mastectomy is more common if the tumor was large, if many nodes (three or more) were involved with cancer, if the tumor had grown into skin or muscle before surgery, or if the margin of the mastectomy was positive.

Radiation therapy greatly reduces the chance that cancer will grow in the area that is radiated. As noted on page 91, radiation therapy after a mastectomy may also reduce the growth of cancer in areas other than where the radiation was given. The theory developed to explain these observations is that some women might not have metastasis from their initial cancer; but if the cancer persists or regrows in the breast area, the women are exposed a second time to the risk that cells might spread from the cancer and grow into metastases. Radiation therapy reduces the chance that cancer will regrow a second time and have a second opportunity to spread.

It is important to emphasize that these studies were done in women with high-risk cancers as shown by the fact that about one-third of the women who did not receive radiation therapy had local recurrence on the chest wall. High local recurrence rates indicate high-risk cancers.

If you had a mastectomy for a large cancer, if the cancer had grown into the skin or muscle, or if many nodes were involved, you will benefit from radiation therapy to your chest wall. There is no consensus on how many nodes need to be involved before recommending radiation therapy. Certainly, if more than three nodes are involved, radiation should be considered. Whether radiation should be recommended when only one or two nodes are involved is still unclear.

Adjuvant Therapy

"Do I need adjuvant therapy?"

    Adjuvant therapy is treatment given to women who have been diagnosed with breast cancer before there is any evidence of further cancer elsewhere in the body.

    Typically adjuvant therapy has been either administration of chemicals that kill cancer cells (called chemotherapy) or use of drugs or surgery to change the hormones in a woman's body (called hormone-based therapy). Recently there are new drugs—*targeted biologic drugs* (page 101)—that target specific steps in cancer growth.

    In general terms, the decision to use chemotherapy and the decision to use hormone-based therapy are very similar with very similar expected benefits. Which treatment to use is influenced by the age of the patient, whether the tumor has hormone receptors, and the degree of danger that the cancer presents. Chemotherapy is typically used for women who are still having regular periods at the time of diagnosis of their cancer, and hormone-based therapy is used for women who have gone through menopause. For higher risk situations—high growth rate, large number of positive nodes, high grade—chemotherapy may be appropriate for postmenopausal women; for lower risk situations, hormone-based therapy may be appropriate for young women who are still menstruating. For some women both may be appropriate.

Chemotherapy

"Do I need chemotherapy?"

    Chemotherapy is the administration of toxic drugs that kill fast-growing cells as they grow. Chemotherapy is given with the understanding that cancer cells will be more vulnerable to the drugs than will normal cells. It is expected for most chemotherapy that there will be side effects on normal cells also; but it is assumed that the benefits in terms of killing cancer cells will outweigh the problems or the side effects of taking the drugs.

    Chemotherapy can make a bad situation better, but it cannot make it perfect. For example, if a woman has several positive nodes and a 3-centimeter cancer, she has about a 50% chance of developing cancer metastases over 10 years. Chemotherapy will reduce this chance of metastases to 35% to 40%. This is an improvement of 10% to 15%.

This 10% to 15% reduction of chance of metastases is about one-quarter of the entire 50% chance of recurrence, i.e., 10% to 15% is about one-quarter of 50%. It is common to say that chemotherapy has reduced the chance of recurrence by a quarter although the real difference is only about 10% to 15%. This is similar to discussions about relative risk and absolute risk. (See page 40.) This reflects the common practice of putting the best possible interpretation on the known results of any therapy.

The effect of chemotherapy is surprisingly similar for many different regimens, and over fairly long periods of time. Chemotherapy will reduce the relative chance of dying over any period of time by about 25%. It is very important to emphasize again that this 25% refers to a quarter of the chance of dying, not to an overall, absolute 25% improvement in survival.

An example of a more favorable tumor will help show how this works. If a woman has a nonaggressive cancer, for example a one-centimeter, grade I cancer with negative nodes, she has only about a 10% chance of metastases over 10 years. If she takes chemotherapy, she will reduce this chance by about a quarter, but since the absolute risk is lower, the absolute reduction will be much lower, i.e., one quarter of 10%, or 2.5%. Stated another way, she will improve her absolute chance of disease-free survival by only about 2.5%. This might have value to a person, but in absolute terms, she will have much less absolute benefit from the chemotherapy than the woman with a more dangerous cancer.

When you decide whether to use chemotherapy, begin by asking your doctor for an estimate of your risk of recurrence. It may be difficult to give a precise number, but it is always possible to say whether the risk is relatively high or low. There is not a medical answer to the question of whether to use chemotherapy in a low-risk situation. If your cancer is low risk, this is your decision.

"What chemotherapy should I have?"

The best chemotherapy has changed since the first edition of this book, and the best choice will *almost certainly change again.* Since the first practical chemotherapy regimen for breast cancer was published in 1976, the overall general evolution of chemotherapy in the United States has been as follows:

- CMF: six monthly cycles of cyclophosphamide, methotrexate, and flouracil
- AC: four cycles of Adriamycin (chemical name doxyrubicin) and cyclophosphamide given every three weeks
- AC-Taxol: four cycles, three weeks apart of AC followed by four cycles of paclitaxel (brand name Taxol)
- Dose Dense AC-T: same drugs given every two weeks using growth factors (see side effects below) to support white blood cells
- Dose Dense AC followed by weekly paclitaxel (Taxol).

Each of these regimens is better tolerated and/or gives slightly better results than its predecessor, but your oncologist may chose a different one for a specific reason for your care.

"What are the side effects of chemotherapy?"

Chemotherapy can cause leukemia or malignant blood diseases. The rate is quite low, about one-quarter of one percent in one study and about half a percent in another, but this is another reason why chemotherapy should only be given if there is a clear benefit that is greater than the risk.

The other major side effects of chemotherapy are caused when the drugs affect normal cells in addition to cancer cells. Nausea, vomiting, hair loss, and low white blood cell counts are to be expected but are usually reversible and go away after therapy is completed.

Side effects are felt most in areas where cells must grow all the time for a given body function to occur. For example, white blood cells must grow all the time to help the body resist infection. *Leucopenia,* or low white blood counts, increases the risk of all infections. Therefore, bioengineered growth factors are often used to force the bone marrow to make adequate white blood cells.

Nausea results from a direct effect of drugs on the *chemotherapy trigger zone,* an area on the brain that controls vomiting. Older drugs had some effects on this brain center, but newer drugs are quite effective in preventing nausea for most women.

Weight gain is common during chemotherapy. This extra weight is often difficult to lose after the end of chemotherapy.

The majority of women experience extensive hair loss after chemotherapy because chemotherapy damages the attachment of the hair root to the hair follicle. A new way to reduce hair loss is for the patient to wear a very cold head cap during chemotherapy. The cap is cold enough to reduce blood flow to the scalp so hair follicles are less exposed to the drugs. This works for many women, but wearing the cold cap can be quite uncomfortable.

Premature menopause is a major risk for women who have chemotherapy. Women who are thrown into menopause by chemotherapy will often experience hot flashes, vaginal dryness, emotional effects of loss of hormones, and secondary effects of hormone loss that can increase osteoporosis. Although some patients have had children years after chemotherapy, it is best to assume that a woman who has chemotherapy will go through menopause and not be able to have more children.

If a woman wants to have children in the future, she should consult with a fertility specialist before starting chemotherapy. There are drugs that may protect the ovaries during chemotherapy, but it is not known how effective they will be for all women. Also, fertility techniques can harvest a woman's eggs before she begins chemotherapy, and those eggs can be frozen for a pregnancy at a future time.

Hormone-Based Therapy

"Do I need hormone-based therapy?"

Hormone-based therapy is an alternative to chemotherapy that is used for women whose cancers would be expected to respond to hormones. Hormone-based therapy helps *only* women with ER and/or PR positive cancers.

The goal of hormone-based therapy is to remove the effects of estrogens. This treats cancer because when cells lose estrogens, they lose activation of estrogen receptors, and they stop growing. This is the opposite of the untreated situation where *estrogens activate the estrogen receptor*, and that activation makes ER positive cells grow.

Estrogens are made in the ovaries of younger women who are still having menstrual periods. For these women, estrogens can be removed literally by removing ovaries surgically, destroying the ovaries with radiation, or turning off the ovaries with LHRH agonists.

However, in premenopausal women, it is much more common to remove estrogens *virtually*, i.e., the hormones are still present, but a drug is given to block the effects of estrogens on cancer cells. The most widely used drug is tamoxifen. There are also newer drugs that block production of estrogens in the ovaries by interfering with normal control of the ovaries by the brain.

In contrast, women who have gone through menopause usually do not make estrogens in their ovaries, but they do make smaller amounts of estrogens in fatty tissue, and small amounts of estrogen can be made in the breast itself. The benefits of hormone-based therapy in women who have gone through menopause are similar to the benefits of chemotherapy for women who are still having regular menstruation when their cancer is diagnosed.

If a tumor has hormone receptors, i.e., the tumor is hormone (estrogen and/or progesterone) receptor *positive*, then hormone therapy will usually be beneficial. If the tumor is small, of low grade, and the nodes are negative, the benefits of hormone-based therapy may be small in absolute terms. However, hormone-based drugs have such mild side effects that that they are usually prescribed for most ER positive cancers.

For women who have tumors that are hormone receptive, there is about a one-quarter reduction in the risk of metastases or death. As with chemotherapy, hormone therapy is more beneficial for women with more dangerous cancers, but there is less absolute benefit for less dangerous cancers.

Adding progestins is a kind of hormone therapy that is occasionally used for advanced cancer. Progestins seem to oppose the effects of estrogens. They can be given as a pill, but there are more side effects of weight gain and nausea with progestins than with estrogen removal.

"What is an aromatase inhibitor?"

To make estrogens, the ovary (or another site) must change the shape of a molecule to include a new chemical ring of carbon atoms. This ring is called an *aromatic ring* because it is an essential part of the chemicals that cause aromas, such as the aroma of strawberries. Because this enzyme used to make estrogen makes an aromatic ring, it is called an *aromatase*.

If the aromatase is inhibited and cannot function, it blocks formation of estrogens. In post-menopausal women, an aromatase inhibitor (AI) gives slightly better statistical survival rates than does tamoxifen.

For premenopausal women, however, AIs often have the opposite effect and stimulate the ovaries. This is why aromatase inhibitors can be used to stimulate egg formation for *in vitro* fertility care, and it is why AIs are *not used* to treat breast cancer in younger women unless the ovaries have totally stopped functioning.

"What are the side effects of hormone therapy?"

The most common effects of estrogen withdrawal or blocking are menopause symptoms. Lack of estrogen causes hot flashes, vaginal dryness or itching, weight gain, and/or unwanted facial hair.

Loss of estrogen by removal of the ovaries—or blocking estrogen formation with an aromatase inhibitor—increases the risk of osteoporosis. In contrast, although tamoxifen blocks the effects of estrogens on cancer cells, it helps maintain bone density and prevent osteoporosis.

The worst side effect of tamoxifen is uterine cancer in a small proportion of women. About 1% of women who take tamoxifen develop uterine cancer they would not otherwise have had. Therefore, when tamoxifen is used, it should be in a situation in which you expect at least 2% or more increase in the chance of survival. Otherwise, the risk from the drug will be the same as the benefit. Tamoxifen has also been implicated in cataracts, retinal damage, and venous thrombosis (blood clots that can lead to life threatening pulmonary embolus).

"How do the side effects of tamoxifen and AIs compare?"

Both tamoxifen and AIs take away estrogen effects. They can both cause vaginal dryness, increased hot flashes, skin dryness, and, for some women, a *cognitive change* that is annoying but very hard to define. The cognitive change usually involves difficulty recalling words and names.

For bones, tamoxifen provides some protection against osteoporosis. AIs do not directly harm bones, but they do predispose a person to osteoporosis and fractures, such as hip fractures. For this reason, some experts prescribe tamoxifen instead of an AI if a woman already has osteroporosis.

For the heart, tamoxifen provides some improvement in cholesterol levels. AIs have the opposite effect.

For the uterus, tamoxifen increases the risk of uterine cancer. AIs decrease the risk of uterine cancer.

For blood clots, tamoxifen increases the risk. AIs decrease the risk.

About 30% of women who take AIs develop a painful muscle-skeletal syndrome of aches. It is claimed that tamoxifen causes the same syndrome, but speaking from personal observation, I have yet to see a woman discontinue tamoxifen because of muscle or skeletal pain.

"How long should I take tamoxifen?"

Two years of tamoxifen is better than no tamoxifen, five years is better than two years, and *ten years treatment with tamoxifen or an aromatase inhibitor is more effective than five years treatment.*

Initially, there was concern that after five years tamoxifen might begin to stimulate growth of cancer rather than suppress growth. However, meta-analysis showed that if tamoxifen is stopped after five years, survival to ten years is the same as if taking tamoxifen the whole ten years. However, if you stopped tamoxifen after five years, survival after ten years, i.e., *between ten and fifteen years from diagnosis, was not as good* as if a patient took tamoxifen for the whole ten years. Thus, the *benefits of tamoxifen last about five years after a person stops taking the drug.*

The absolute benefit from tamoxifen drops over time because the risk of recurrence drops over time, but unfortunately, the *side effects of tamoxifen do not decrease over time.* For bad cancers, one would probably take tamoxifen for a long time because the late risk is higher than for less dangerous cancers. However, for less dangerous cancers, there is probably a time when the risk of side effects becomes greater than any benefit.

"How long should I take an aromatase inhibitor?"

A preliminary report has found a similar benefit from ten years of an aromatase inhibitor rather than just five years. This is good for many women, but the risks in terms of arthritis and osteoporosis must be balanced against the diminishing absolute benefit. Again, longer treatment makes sense for more difficult cancers.

"Should I use both chemotherapy and hormone-based therapy?"

Women who take tamoxifen in addition to chemotherapy have increased survival, if they have hormone receptor positive cancers. The benefit from tamoxifen is less than the benefit from chemotherapy, i.e., the chemotherapy will reduce recurrence by about one-quarter to one-third, but tamoxifen in addition to chemotherapy adds only about half that benefit. When the benefit is very small, it may not be worthwhile to add tamoxifen.

However, the opposite is also be true. For a small, strongly ER positive tumor, the *benefit of hormone treatment by itself may be sufficient that chemotherapy does not add significant benefit.* The 21-gene and 70-gene assays are often used to support this recommendation.

"What is targeted biologic therapy?"

Targeted biologic therapy means that a drug is directed at one specific step or set of steps in the metabolism of cancer. In one sense, hormone-based therapy (page 97) is a targeted biologic therapy because it targets the action of the estrogen receptor. However, hormone-based therapy (in its original form as removal of ovaries to stop estrogen production) has been around for more than 100 years—preceding chemotherapy by half a century—so it is considered a separate kind of therapy by itself.

"What is trastuzumab?"

Trastuzumab (brand name, Herceptin) is the first targeted biologic therapy to be used widely and successfully.

About 20% of invasive ductal breast cancers have excessive HER2 receptors on the surface of most of the cancer cells. When this receptor is activated, it makes the cancer grow aggressively. Trastuzumab—which is given as an injection every few weeks—blocks the HER2 receptor. When the receptor is blocked, the cells grow more slowly or stop growing all together.

Trastuzumab generally has few side effects. However, the HER2 receptor is also on muscle cells in the heart, and about one percent of women who take the drug will have reduced heart function. Usually the heart recovers when the drug is discontinued.

"Are there other drugs that target the HER2 receptors?"

Lapatinib is a pill, rather than an injection, that is used to block the function of the HER2 receptor. Lapatinib has limited use because of significant side effects. Pertuzumab is a newer drug—also given by injection—that complements the action of trastuzumab. Trastuzumad and pertuzumab are often given together. TDM1 is a different strategy that links a strong chemotherapy drug to trastuzumab so the drug is carried specifically to cancer cells where the anti-HER2 antibody binds to HER2 positive cells bringing the drug with it. This is an area of active research. Ask your physician for the most recent information.

"What are other targeted therapies to treat breast cancer?"

If you have metastatic cancer, you may be treated with a new group of drugs that target individual genes in cancer cells. (Technically, these drugs sometimes target the gene and sometimes target the protein made by the gene.) These drugs focus on specific steps in cancer metabolism.

A non-cancerous cell does not convert to a cancer cell in one step. *Many things must change in a cell for it to become cancerous.* Usually this means that the actions of many genes are changed. Typically, changes affect steps in a *metabolic pathway.* Newer drugs *target these changes individually,* i.e., one at a time.

"What is a metabolic pathway?"

A metabolic pathway is a set of genes and proteins that work in a sequence of steps to make things happen in the life of a cell. You can think of a *pathway like a series of dominoes where one step tips off the next step, that tips the next step, etc.* (Technically, its a series of genes that encode for proteins, and each protein activates—or in some cases inactivates—either the gene or the protein for the next step in the pathway.)

Most of the steps in a pathway make the pathway active, but some stop the pathway from acting. PTEN and p53 are important genes that stop cell growth and facilitate cell death by stopping a metabolic pathway. The outcome of a pathway depends on the balance between the genes that make it active and the genes that slow it down.

"What is the mTOR pathway?"

Most cancer cells use a metabolic pathway called the PI3K/ AKT/ mTOR pathway or sometimes simply the mTOR pathway. When the mTOR pathway is *activated*, cells make new DNA so they can divide into more cells, and they resist dying.

While the PI3K/ AKT/ mTOR pathway makes cells grow and resist cell death, two companion genes—PTEN and p53—slow or block the same pathway. The genes that block the pathway are as important as the genes that activate the pathway. They all contribute to the *balance that determines* what will happen. Pathways are sometimes drawn with arrows to show what gene triggers what other genes.

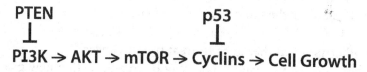

PTEN   p53

⊥   ⊥

PI3K → AKT → mTOR → Cyclins → Cell Growth

The arrow (->) means the first gene activates the next gene. The upside down T means this gene blocks the gene or action at the end of the upside down T.

"How do biologic drugs treat cancer?"

New biologic drugs work by interrupting specific, individual steps of the mTOR pathway. Since this is such a central pathway in the growth of cells, *loss of any step in this pathway will stop the whole pathway* and inhibit the growth of cells.

Currently, there are drugs that block mTOR directly by itself (everolimus), cyclins directly by themselves (palbociclib) and PI3K directly by itself. These drugs can be beneficial but they can also have serious side effects, so they are currently restricted to use for advanced cancer.

This is an exciting change from 40 years ago when the available drugs either poisoned cancer cells—and a lot of normal cells, too—or blocked estrogens. Future research will discover whether these are the best biologic drugs, or if there are others that work better and/or with fewer side effects.

"Should I join a clinical trial?"

Physicians can only learn how to use a new drug, or an old drug in a new way, by the results of clinical trials. Note that I specify drugs, but a *clinical trial may also apply to any kind of treatment* such as the clinical trials that demonstrated that mastectomy is not necessary for many women or the clinical trials showing the benefit of mammograms to screen for breast cancer. Clinical trial means that the drug or treatment was tested with real people, in the clinic, so to speak.

For a *clinical trial*, a woman consents to take an experimental drug (or an existing drug used in a new way). Typically a clinical trial makes a comparison between two drugs, or one drug and a placebo (a non-active "sugar pill"). The decision of which drug a woman receives is made by chance (randomized) by the study center and is out of the control of the woman's personal physician (page 19).

Clinical trials usually focus on specific groups of patients and test specific comparisons of drugs. The appendix gives a list of examples of recently published clinical trials that have helped guide treatment of many women.

If you have a cancer with a proven, established treatment, then you may not be appropriate for a clinical trial. However, sometimes there is valid reason to think that a new treatment may give better results than what would be available from usual treatment. In that case, you may benefit from entering a clinical trial. Signing up for a clinical trial is 100% your decision. A clinical trial is only appropriate if there is no basis to know if one treatment or the other is better.

Family Issues: Talking to Your Children, Family Planning, Female Relatives

"What do I say to my children?"

Children, especially young children, perceive your anxiety, probably long before you admit to yourself that you are scared. Your cancer is a very threatening disruption in their lives. They will feel insecure, doubt your love for them, and wonder if you are going to leave or abandon them. The smaller the child, the more these fears will give them anxiety about their own survival, but even older children will have these fears. Small children will more often than not assume that they have, in some way, caused the problem unless you explain to them otherwise.

The best plan is to be open and honest and to let your children know what is causing your preoccupation. If they know what the cause of your concern is, *and that it is not them*, they will begin to understand that you still love and will care for them. Your feelings toward them are the key. Take extra time to assure your children that the problem is not something they caused, and that you still love them. It is not necessary, and it may be unwise to be so explicit as to say that you are scared of dying; but it is better to allow your children to know that you are scared than to let them imagine that in some way you are angry with them. Ask for professional help from the various groups that are ready to help you. (See Resources on page 112.)

"Can I ever take hormones or birth control pills again?"

Estrogens are the basis of menopausal hormone replacement therapy as well as the basis of most birth control pills or oral contraceptives. Estrogens are important for breast growth, and estrogens will make breast tissue grow in women who have gone through menopause, adolescents, and even men. Removing estrogens is also known to be beneficial for the treatment of many breast cancers.

Logic would seem to indicate that if adding estrogens makes breasts grow, and taking away estrogens makes breast tissue stop growing, then giving estrogens must be bad for women who have breast cancer. As clever as this logic is, it is not proven. It is simply something for which physicians don't really have an answer and therefore they, as a group, take the stand that seems to be most cautious. This does not mean that it is OK to take estrogens or birth control pills. It means that no one knows if it is safe or not. Menopause can be a very difficult experience. It can be especially difficult for young women who experience menopause because of chemotherapy.

In informal discussions with colleagues, I cannot find an oncologist who has not prescribed estrogens for a woman who has had cancer. They prescribed estrogens because the effects of menopause, either symptoms or bone loss, were severe enough to justify the risk that the estrogen might actually make the cancer worse. In each case it has been with much reluctance and many cautions that this is an unproven step that may cause harm. It is important to recognize, however, that as bad as cancer can be, life must also be pleasant enough to be worth living.

"How does breast cancer relate to pregnancy?"

Breast cancer can relate to pregnancy in three ways, depending on the timing of the pregnancy and the cancer. These situations are very different in their potential to affect a woman's health. Thus it is important to specify exactly the question that is being asked.

In one situation, a *woman who has gone through breast cancer* wonders if she will risk her health to have a child.

In the second situation, *a woman is pregnant* and learns that she has breast cancer. (Fortunately, less than one percent of breast cancer in young women occurs in women who are pregnant.)

In the third situation, a *woman has recently had a baby* and learns that she has breast cancer.

"Is it safe to have a baby if I've had breast cancer?"

The traditional teaching was that a woman who has had breast cancer should never consider having a baby. It was assumed that the high hormone levels of pregnancy would stimulate the growth of any remnant of cancer that might be left behind. This assumption was based on the observation that women who are pregnant when they develop breast cancer have a poorer prognosis than those who are not. This observation is true, but the poor prognosis probably results from the combination of delayed diagnosis and likely different breast cancer biology.

Breasts change a lot during pregnancy. There are frequent cysts in the breast during pregnancy, that often resolve on their own. In many cases, pregnant women who have breast cancer are reassured, *incorrectly*, by their physician that what is actually cancer is "just a cyst." These women are sometimes untreated for the duration of pregnancy or even a period of breast-feeding. This leads to a worse prognosis and may explain why it seems that women who are pregnant when they discover breast cancer do less well than women who are not pregnant.

Many studies have found that pregnancy after breast cancer does not make cancer worse ###. These studies have compared the experience of women who became pregnant to women with similar cancers who did not become pregnant. When they compared similar types of tumors, there was similar outcome whether or not a woman became *pregnant after her breast cancer.*

"What do I do if I get breast cancer *during pregnancy?*"

Breast cancer during a woman's pregnancy is usually treated based on the stage of the pregnancy.

The fetus is most vulnerable during the first trimester (the first 14 weeks of the pregnancy) and neither general anesthesia nor drugs are recommended during that time. Local anesthesia for a biopsy is generally safe.

There is good experience that surgery can be done during the second trimester of pregnancy (from week 14 through week 28). Also, some chemotherapy drugs can be given during the second trimester. It is usually best to work not only with your oncologist but also a specialist in high-risk pregnancies.

Hormone-acting therapy cannot be used during pregnancy, and most physicians try to avoid radiation therapy, although it has been used during pregnancy.

The challenges of breast cancer during pregnancy are mostly the logistics of finding treatment that will not harm the fetus.

Breast cancer is not a specific reason to terminate a pregnancy.

"Is it worse if I get breast cancer right after a pregnancy?"

There is debate whether the biology of breast cancer is worse if the cancer develops during or in the first few years after pregnancy, compared with non-pregnancy-associated cancer. The earlier belief was that the poorer prognosis for pregnancy-associated cancer was because of failure to recognize and diagnose the cancer. More recently, however, researchers have come to believe that pregnancy-associated breast cancer has a different biology.

The breast grows during pregnancy, and the factors that cause growth of the breast for nursing might also make breast cancer more likely to develop and possibly be more aggressive. There is stronger evidence that breast cancer developing in the first several years *after pregnancy* is more aggressive (than non-pregnancy-associated cancer), than evidence that breast cancer developing *during pregnancy* is more aggressive.

It is important to note, however, that not all studies find a worse prognosis when breast cancer is associated with pregnancy.

"What should my daughter, sister, mother do?"

Your cancer does not cause anyone else to be at higher risk.

People who share your genetic heritage (that is, your blood relatives) share a similar risk to yours. If you have cancer, the risk has become a reality for you. Your relatives' risk does not change because you have had cancer.

The reply to relatives should be that because they share your heritage they may have inherited a risk themselves. Knowledge of your cancer constitutes a warning that they, too, might be at more-than-average risk. They should take good care of themselves, be familiar with their own breasts, do breast self-examination, have appropriate mammograms, and see a health professional regularly to check their own health. With luck, they will never experience cancer; but if they do, it is neither your fault nor theirs. Guidelines for their self-care are discussed in Parts One and Two. Remember, most daughters of women with breast cancer *do not develop breast cancer.*

Taking Control

"What should I do when I leave your office?"

YOU HAVE TIME!

The best available evidence is that you have can wait at least 4 weeks from biopsy, and probably up to 90 days, without a worse outcome. A delay of more than 90 days may be harmful, but even that is only a minor change as long as a woman will be taking either a hormone-based therapy or chemotherapy. Delays of 6 months or longer are likely to reduce survival.

Cancer is virtually always unexpected, even for a woman who has considered herself to be at high risk. The most important thing to do is to ask questions and to learn. Keep a paper and pen handy to write down questions as they come to mind. This will allow you to remember your questions for the next time you see your physician, and it will relieve you of the anxiety of trying to remember what you want to ask.

Think through whom you believe you can ask for help. Ask a friend to go with you to physician visits to help you remember what was said or take notes for you. Record conversations with your physicians.

Ask your physician for people to talk with. Seek counsel from your clergy, a counselor, or a wise friend. Don't be afraid to ask. Don't be afraid to be honest with those you feel you can trust.

"Would a therapist be helpful?"

Breast cancer causes a time of great stress. There is threat to life and there is usually at least some change in one's perception of self. These stresses can sometimes be handled by conversation with friends or other women who have had cancer. Sometimes the stress is more severe.

Breast cancer for some women is a wake-up call that life is not an inexhaustible resource. Sometimes there are problems that have been deferred or which seemed less important if one were thinking only about career, family, etc. Cancer will bring these problems to the forefront, and if it has been uncomfortable to think about them before, it will not be any easier now. For these reasons, it is often useful to speak with someone who is a professional counselor. A clergy person, a wise mentor, or a psychotherapist might be helpful. It is useful if this person has some understanding of cancer. Most often, if you have health insurance, it will cover support of this kind. Also, many hospitals and community groups sponsor free or sliding-scale groups for women diagnosed with breast cancer.

"What should I do next week, next month, next year?"

You can take some time to decide what you want to do. There is good data from observation of women who were treated more than 20 years ago that you can take at least up to 4 weeks between a biopsy and the next steps in treatment. Similarly, there is some evidence that a delay of *over 90 days* may be harmful, Now is the time to get as many opinions as you need to become satisfied that you are able to make a choice that feels right for you.

It is better to take a few extra days now to learn more, than to run to some treatment plan and have to wonder a month or a year from now if you did the right thing. Go ahead when you are ready, but it is best to go ahead within no longer than 12 weeks.

For the next several months take special care of yourself. Let your spouse, lover, friends and relatives help you. Surgery, anesthesia, radiation therapy, chemotherapy, and even worry will take energy. Your body needs rest to recover. You will not be able to work full time and have a busy social life. You will need more rest than usual. This is a temporary time, but you will recover much more quickly if you rest when you need it.

Exercise is an important way to recover and preserve your strength. Unused muscles rapidly lose strength, and you are likely to be old enough (older than 30) that regaining muscle strength is a long, painful process. It is better to protect your muscles and strength as you go along. Muscles respond to use, so use your muscles.

If you are tired, walk and then rest. Don't just sit in a chair and not walk. It is more beneficial to walk for 15 minutes and sleep for 2 hours than to sit up for 2 hours. The important time is the time you use your muscles!

A good diet is also important, but avoid hypervitaminosis (taking too many vitamins), which can interfere with healing. High doses of vitamin E can slow healing. High doses of vitamin C can help. Talk to your physician about all vitamins and herbs you use. Vitamin A is also useful for healing, but high doses can damage your liver if taken for more than two or three weeks.

Over the next years you will need to work with your physician to watch how you respond to therapy and to be certain there are not other problems. It is an unfortunate fact that some women who have breast cancer will have a recurrence; and metastasis is a major threat to life.

There are several other risks. Cancer in the opposite breast is a real risk and a woman should have annual mammograms of her other breast and a careful examination at least yearly or perhaps more often. Increased ovarian cancer (and to a lesser extent colon and uterine cancer) are somewhat associated with breast cancer, and a woman should have a gynecological evaluation by her gynecologist, her primary physician or her oncologist on a regular basis.

Many tests have been proposed for the detection of recurrent breast cancer. In general, they do not really help. If tests are negative, it does not prove there is no possibility of a problem. Randomized trials have shown that women who come to their physician when they have a concern do just as well as women who have many routine tests. Most experts agree that a yearly mammogram of the opposite breast will help detect a new cancer earlier than otherwise, but a set of routine tests, scans, etc., will not improve survival. Breast self-examination is helpful but should be in addition to, not a substitute for, careful follow-up.

The best solution for long-term care is to have a good working relationship with your breast care physician. This can be your surgeon, your oncologist, your radiation oncologist, or your primary physician. It should be a person who is knowledgeable and experienced in following women who have had breast cancer. *You are seeking a person who has a good sense of what to expect and who will be well attuned to detecting deviations from what is expected.*

"Who will take care of me next? What are their qualifications?"

Care of breast cancer involves many types of specialists. The value of specialists is that they have a wide range of experience and will be more sensitive to detecting when something is not going as planned. They will also have a better sense of when everything is going as expected.

For chemotherapy and radiation therapy, it is important to have a specially trained oncologist. If surgery is required, you want a person who has adequate experience and who has done many breast operations.

BEYOND THIS BOOK

Physicians function in society as the people who study health and disease and seek ways to use this information to inform and to treat patients. From a sociological perspective they have an unwritten but clearly accepted duty to be as objective and as free from bias as possible in this role.

Once we are certain of the actual causes of cancer, we will have an opportunity to set goals for the prevention of cancer. It is important, however, to be cautious about assuming that something that seems obvious is the real answer. As a nation, we seem to want to have quick answers that point to other people. This desire for *quick* answers creates a risk that we will overlook or miss the *real* answer. Then we could make many changes with no real benefit.

The setting of priorities within the United States is responsive to the interests of those who advocate for various causes. Breast cancer is a major cause of poor health and death for American women; yet, on a personal note, 25 years ago, the then-dean of a major medical school advised me that it was a dead-end field.

The answers to questions explained in this book represent the collective histories of millions of women. They also represent the dedication of many physicians, research scientists, and advocates, and, most importantly, the contributions of women who allowed themselves to be subjects for the scientific studies of breast cancer. This book is an introduction to their collective histories.

Your opportunity now is to give active support to those who speak for improved understanding of breast cancer. Speak for improved care of yourself. Participate in clinical trials, if appropriate. Participate in the creation of the recorded complex history of breast cancer so that other women can benefit from your experience. Speak for yourself.

INFORMATION RESOURCES

American Cancer Society (www.cancer.org) A resource for the general public.

Army of Women (www.armyofwomen.org) Dr. Susan Love's Army of Women dedicated to finding the cause of breast cancer.

Brainmetsbc(www.brainmetsbc.org) Resource for understanding brain metastases, treatments and the latest research.

Breast Cancer Action (www.bcaction.org) National grassroots organization challenging the status quo and working to address and end the breast cancer epidemic.

Breast Cancer Fund (http://www.breastcancerfund.org) San Francisco breast cancer organization focused on prevention and improved treatment of breast cancer.

Drugs used to treat breast cancer (www.breastcancer.org/treatment/druglist) Useful list of drugs used to treat breast cancer discussing their side effects.

Environmental Working Group (www.EWG.org) National group advocating a safer environment for all of us. A *leader in identifying risks* from personal care products and food contaminants. Publishes online *lists of safer cosmetic and personal care products.*

Fertile Hope (www.fertilehope.org) Fertility issues in women with breast cancer.

FORCE (www.facingourrisk.org) Resource for women at high risk for breast cancer for support and current information.

Inflammatory Breast Cancer (www.ibcsupport.org) Provides accurate and helpful information for patients with IBC.

Living with Breast Cancer (www.breastcancer.org) Website created by Dr. Marisa Weiss, a radiation oncologist.

Metastatic Breast Cancer Information and Support (www.bcmets.org) Provides a list of services for women with metastatic breast cancer.

National Breast Cancer Coalition (www.stopbreastcancer.org) a national organization focused on political and policy issues.

National Cancer Institute (www.cancer.gov) A comprehensive resource for both doctors and patients. Clinical trials are included as well.

Nation Cancer Institute Designated Cancer Centers (www.cancercenters.cancer.gov) Lists the NCI Designated Cancer Centers by State.

National Center for Complementary and Alternative Medicine (www.nccam.nih.gov)
Resource for scientific information on complementary and alternative therapies.

National Comprehensive Cancer Network (www.nccn.com) A resource to help patients navigate through their experience with cancer and to know the practice guidelines dealing with breast cancer.

National Lymphedema Network (www.lymphnet.org) Resource for lymphedema caused by breast cancer.

PubMed (http://www.ncbi.nlm.nih.gov/pubmed) The National Library of Medicine at the National Institute of Health. **The absolute best source of up to date current research on breast cancer and any other health issue.** Provides free abstracts of almost all articles, and many practice-changing articles can be downloaded free of charge.

Y-ME (www.y-me.org) Provides information for clinical questions and support for women diagnosed with breast cancer (800-221-2141).
Young Survival Coalition (www.youngsurvival.org) Focuses on young women diagnosed and living after their breast cancer treatment.

Zero Breast Cancer (http://www.zerobreastcancer.org) A breast cancer organization focused on Marin County near San Francisco where the rate of breast cancer has been higher.

Medical Complaints in California
Medical Board of California
1-800-633-2322
California Department of Corporations
HMO Complaint Line
1-800-400-0815

Tell Washington:

White House Hotline
202-456-1111

House and Senate Main Switchboard
202-224-3121

EXAMPLES OF NAMING OF CLINICAL TRIALS GROUPS AND RECENT CLINICAL TRIALS

This is not a complete list of clinical trials. It is a representative sample to illustrate how trials are named and how most trials address one question at a time.

AMAROS (2014) – **A**fter **M**apping of the **A**xilla, **R**adiation **or S**urgery? For patients who have a mastectomy and a sentinel node biopsy—and the sentinel node is positive—compared surgery to remove more nodes versus radiation therapy to treat the other nodes. Slightly more lymphedema after axillary dissection. Slightly poorer arm motion after radiation therapy.

ATAC (2010) – **A**rimidex (anastrozole) or **T**amoxifen **A**lone or in **C**ombination. Compared adjuvant use of these drugs along or in combination. Less recurrence with adjuvant anastrozole, but more osteoporosis and not clear if survival difference.

BIG 1-98 – **B**reast **I**nternational **G**roup trial 1-98. For women with estrogen receptor positive breast cancer—with either positive or negative nodes—five years of letrozole gave better survival than five years of tamoxifen. Interestingly, both two years of tamoxifen then switching to letrozole, and two years of letrozole then switching to tamoxifen, were also better than five years tamoxifen and neither was significantly different from five years letrozole alone. There are other BIG trials.

BOLERO (2016) – **B**reast Cancer Trials of **O**ral Everlimus. A set of trials showing some benefit from the mTOR inhibitor, everolimus, in combination with various drugs for metastatic breast cancer, i.e., with trastuzumab and paclitaxel for HER2 positive cancers with exemestane for ER positive cancers, etc.

CLEOPATRA (2015) – **C**linical **E**valuation **of P**ertuzumab and **T**raztuzumab. Found that adding pertuzumab to docetaxel and traztuzumab was superior for metastatic HER2 positive breast cancer.

ECOG (2008) - Eastern Cooperative Oncology Group. Many trials. One key trial demonstrated that weekly paclitaxel (brand name Taxol) is superior both to paclitaxel every three weeks, and to docetaxel (brand name Taxotere) either weekly or every three weeks for both breast cancer survival and overall survival. This trial was in cooperation with SWOG (Southwest Oncology Group), CALGB (Cancer and Leukemia Group B), and NCCTG (North Central Cancer Treatment Group).
Another ECOG trial (2015) found that premenopausal women with a low 21-gene score had very high survival even without chemotherapy.

HERA – Herceptin Adjuvant. Compared two- to one-year of adjuvant Herceptin (trastuzumab). One was as good as two years.

I-SPY (2016) - Investigation of Serial Studies to Predict Your Therapeutic Response with Imaging and Molecular Analysis. This is a modification of a randomized trial called *adaptive design*. The I-SPY trials compare neoadjuvant treatments given before surgery. Patients receive standard therapy plus an experimental therapy. Adaptive design means that adjustments are made in the way drugs are given - during the study - so that promising drugs are tested more thoroughly and less promising drugs are dropped. This design has demonstrated a benefit of adding a new kind of drug, neratinib, to standard therapy for HER2 positive, ER negative, PR negative breast cancer, and velaparib for triple negative breast cancer.

KEYNOTE-012 (2016) - I cannot find the specific meaning of this acronym, but it is likely derived from Keytruda, the brand name for pembroclizumab. The multiple Keynote studies use pembroclizumab to neutralize PD-1 (programmed [cell] death-1) a protein cancers use to suppress natural immunity to the cancer. These studies might make immunotherapy feasible, and there is preliminary evidence that blocking PD-1 may treat triple negative breast cancer. Careful follow up is warranted to see it this becomes a useful treatment.

NSABP (multiple years) – National Surgical Adjuvant Breast (and Bowel) Project. An organization in Pittsburg, PA that has conducted an admirable series of randomized trials of treatment for breast cancer (and more recently bowel cancer).

The studies are numbered in the order they began: B-04 showed it was unnecessary to remove axillary nodes to treat breast cancer (page 91). B-06 showed that long-term survival after breast-conserving surgery was as good as after mastectomy (page 84). B-14 showed that tamoxifen reduced recurrence of breast cancer (page 97). B-18 demonstrated the safety of neoadjuvant chemotherapy to reduce cancer size before surgery (page 87). B-24 showed that tamoxifen reduced future cancer after diagnosis of DCIS (page 73). P-01 showed that tamoxifen reduced future breast cancer rates in women at high risk (page 46).

PALOMA (2015) – PALOMA is a trial of **P**alboclibin and **L**etrozole in **O**estrogen Receptor Positive **M**etastatic **A**denocarcinoma (note that the English spell estrogen with an "O" as *oestrogen*), so the acronym is probably something like that. The trial is the first to show that the CDK4/6 inhibitor palbociclib increases the benefit of letrozole for metastatic breast cancer. PALOMA uses different combinations of drugs, e.g., replacing letrozole with fulvestrant in part 3 of the trial, which may explain the decision not to explain the acronym.

POEMS (2015) - **P**revention **o**f **E**arly **M**enopause **S**tudy found that use of a gonadotropin-releasing hormone (GnRH) agonist drug during chemotherapy reduced the risk that chemotherapy would put a woman into menopause and prevent future pregnancy. GnRH agonists block ovary function temporarily and reversibly by stopping the hormone signals from the brain that normally cause menstruation.

SOFT (2016) – **S**uppression **o**f Ovarian **F**unction **T**rial. Published in a single paper with the TEXT Trial. Evaluated drugs that suppress ovarian function in premenopausal women with ER and/or PR positive and HER2 negative breast cancers. Found added benefit from suppressing ovary function for women at higher risk (who received chemotherapy) on the basis of younger age, more positive nodes, lower ER and PR values (though still positive), higher Ki-67, higher tumor grade, and/or larger tumor size.

STAR (2010) – **S**tudy of **T**amoxifen **a**nd **R**aloxifene. Compared tamoxifen and raloxifene for prevention of breast cancer. Raloxifene is slightly less effective preventing invasive cancer and 25% less effective preventing non-invasive cancer, e.g., DCIS; but significantly fewer side effects of uterine cancer and blood clots.

TAILORx (2015, first part only) – Trial Assigning Individualized Options for Treatment (Rx). Really two trials using the OncoType Recurrence Score to predict the value of adding chemotherapy to hormone-based treatment for women with hormone receptor positive cancers and negative nodes. For women with a Recurrence Score of 10 or less, hormone-based therapy alone gave such good results that chemotherapy would not be recommended. Women with a Recurrence Score of 11 to 26 have received hormone-based treatment and also been randomized to receive chemotherapy or not. These results will be available soon.

TEXT (2016) – Tamoxifen and exemestane Trial See SOFT Trial.

Z-11 (often pronounced "zee eleven") – American College of Surgeons Oncology Group (ACOSOG) Trial Z-011. For women thought to have negative nodes before surgery, but who actually had positive sentinel node(s) when the pathologist examined the node in the laboratory, this study found that doing more surgery to remove additional nodes did not improve survival compared with simple breast radiation and adjuvant therapy, as would be given for the positive lymph node anyway.

GLOSSARY WITH INDEX TO USE IN TEXT

21-gene score – A test done on a sample from a cancer that measures the activity of 21 genes representing hormone receptors, HER2, and growth rates, and calculates a proprietary score that predicts the benefit of chemotherapy assuming that a hormone-based therapy is also used. (p 81)

70-gene signature –A test done on a sample of a cancer that uses the activity of 70 genes to predict whether the cancer has a high or low risk of recurrence. (p 81)

Absolute risk – The difference when the risk in one group (as percent) is subtracted from the risk in another group (as a percent). Technically, this is really the *absolute difference* in risk or difference in absolute risk, but it is customary to drop the word *difference* and say "Absolute Risk." (p 40)

Adjuvant therapy – Drugs, hormones, radiation therapy or other treatment given before there is any evidence of recurrence of cancer. Adjuvant therapy is usually given when the risk of recurrence is considered high. *High* is always a subjective term that you should discuss with your physician. (p 94)

Aromatase inhibitor – A category of drugs that stop the production of estrogen. Cannot be used to treat breast cancer in premenopausal women. (p 98)

Atypical hyperplasia (either ductal or lobular) – A specific subset of fibrocystic change (FCC) in which breast cells that are not cancer grow in a very specific abnormal way. Women who have atypical hyperplasia have an increased risk of developing breast cancer in the next 20 years. About 5% of fibrocystic change has atypical hyperplasia. (p 167)

Axilla/axillary – The area under the arm, or the "armpit." The most common location of lymph nodes related to the breast. Also, the location of the uppermost part of the breast. (p 88)

Basal Cells – Ducts (milk-carrying tubes in the breast) are lined by two layers of cells. The cells farther from the hole in the middle of a duct are called basal cells. These cells give rise to basal type breast cancer. Basal breast cancer (also called triple negative) is the most dangerous type. (p 71 and 80)

Biopsy – Removal of tissue or a sample of tissue from the breast for examination under a microscope by a pathologist. (p 62)

Benign – Not cancerous, not malignant. (p 64)

Bi-Rads – A set of numbers used by radiologists as a standardized scale to indicate how likely it is that a mammogram has identified cancer. Bi-Rads 1 is normal. Bi-Rads 5 is virtually certain to be cancer. (p 36)

Bone scan – A test to look for signs of cancer metastases in bones. A radioactive isotope or chemical is injected into the blood. This isotope is picked up by bones. The scan "camera" looks for abnormal collections of isotopes. Less radiation exposure than taking regular X-rays of all bones. (p 83)

BRCA1 and BRCA2 - Genes necessary to prevent breast cancer. When these genes do not function because of a gene mutation, their failure allows more breast cancer to happen. BRCA 1 and 2 mutations do not actively cause cancer. Rather, they fail to prevent cancer by failing to repair gene damage that happens all the time in everyone. (p 43)

Breast Density – How much the tissue in the breast blocks the X-rays used to make a mammogram. A dense breast contains more water and gland tissue and stops more X-rays so the image is lighter (closer to white) in those areas. (p 43)

Breast Self-Examination (BSE) – A self-administered procedure in which a woman systematically feels her breasts seeking any area that might be cancer. (p 37)

Calcification – A small spot of calcium deposited by the body in the breast and seen on a mammogram. Calcification is a non-specific process that represents an irritation in a focal area. This focal area may or may not be cancer, and a biopsy is often required to find out. (p 35)

c-*erb*-b2 – See HER2.

Chemotherapy – Use of toxic chemicals to kill cancer cells. These chemicals are either injected into the blood or taken as pills. (p 94)

Computerized axial tomography (CAT scan) – A computerized X-ray machine that creates images of focal areas of the body. An excellent test to seek metastases in the lungs or liver. (p 83)

Concordance – A word meaning that the results of two tests agree and give the same answer and that each answer makes sense relative to the other answer. (p 65)

Core biopsy – A way to put a needle through the skin to remove a tiny strip of tissue from a mass or other area that has either been felt or seen with imaging or both. (p 65)

Cyst – Collection of fluid in the breast. Not usually associated with cancer but may be. (p 63)

Cyst aspiration – A way to put a needle through the skin to remove fluid from a cyst. (p 63)

Cytology – Specialized study of individual cells and collections of cells to determine whether cancer is present; the diagnosis of cancer by the study of individual cells. This is familiar to many women because it is similar to the Pap smear used by gynecologists to screen for cervical cancer. (p 63)

Duct/ ductal – The tubes that carry milk from the various parts of the breast to the nipple. The ducts are a network of tubes in all women's breasts. Most breast cancers are thought to start in the ends of the ducts. (p 71)

Ductal carcinoma *in situ* (DCIS) – An *in situ* cancer that is associated with a high risk of invasive cancer developing in the same part of the same breast. (p 72)

Estrogen – A hormone that stimulates development of the breasts and other female characteristics. Thought to protect against heart disease and osteoporosis. Made by the ovaries, the adrenal glands, fatty tissue in general, especially in women (or men) who are overweight, and in small amounts directly in the breast. In general terms, estrogens stimulate the growth of many breast cancers. (p 51)

Estrogen receptor (ER) – See Hormone receptors.

Fibroadenoma – A benign breast tumor that occurs most often in young women but may also occur after menopause. (p 67)

Fibrocystic change – A term used by pathologists to describe a series of changes often seen in breast tissue from women any time in life after adolescence. Fibrocystic change can only be diagnosed by a biopsy. Fibrocystic change occurs in most women by mid-life. Most fibrocystic change does not indicate an increased risk of developing breast cancer. (p 54) See Atypical hyperplasia.

Fibrocystic disease – See Fibrocystic change. Sometimes used to describe what a physician feels on breast examination. The term "fibrocystic disease" should be avoided because it *has no reliable meaning* if the "diagnosis" is based on examination alone. (p 54)

Fine needle aspiration (FNA) – Use of a small needle to remove cells from a breast mass. The cytology of these cells is studied to determine if the mass is cancer or if it is benign. (p 63)

Genetic testing – Laboratory testing that looks at cells (blood, cells in saliva, or cells from another source) to determine whether the person has inherited a change in their genes (a mutation) that impairs the function of a vital gene. Can test not only for genes that cause cancer but also for other diseases. (p 43)

Grade – A term used to describe the combined characteristics of a cancer as seen under a microscope by a pathologist. High-grade cancers are more dangerous than low-grade cancers. (p 77)

HER2 – A gene that codes for a specific receptor (p185), which may be abundant on the surface of individual cancer cells. Cancers that have more HER2 are more dangerous, but they also seem to respond to the antibodies trastuzumab and pertuzumab. HER2 is also referred to as HER2/neu and c-erb-b2. (p 79)

HER2/neu – See HER2.

Histology – Study of tissue removed by biopsy or other surgery to determine whether it is or is not cancer. Histology looks at cytology and the overall structure of the tissue to determine whether cancer is present. (p 65)

Hormone receptors – Specialized proteins on and in cells that, when exposed to hormones such as estrogen and progesterone, cause changes inside the cells that make the cells grow. Tests for hormone receptors help physicians anticipate whether drugs that prevent the actions of hormones will be successful in treating a cancer. (p 79)

Hormone-based therapy – Therapy to decrease the effects of estrogens on hormone receptors. Hormone therapy includes drugs that block estrogen hormone receptors (e.g., tamoxifen or raloxifene), removal of sources of hormones (e.g., surgical removal of ovaries), addition of excess progesterone, drugs that prevent the body from making estrogens, or addition of extremely strong estrogens (which surprisingly work for some women). (p 97)

Hyperplasia – Also called proliferative fibrocystic change. Overgrowth of a tissue or the cells in a tissue. In the breast, usually refers to increased growth of the cells that normally grow inside the ducts of the breast. (p 67)

Inflammatory breast cancer – An aggressive form of cancer that makes the breast look red and swollen as though it was inflamed by an infection. Sometimes mistaken for an infection. (p 76)

In situ cancer – Cancer composed of cells that are growing without the body's normal controls but that have not yet developed the ability to make their own space, attract new blood vessels to themselves, and invade tissue outside of gland tissue in the breast. *In situ* cancer cannot yet grow outside of the breast, and it usually cannot cause death unless it changes and becomes invasive cancer. (p 70)

Invasive cancer – Cancer composed of cells that can destroy and make their own space in normal tissue and can attract new blood vessels to support their own growth. Invasive cancer can grow outside of the breast, become metastatic, and cause death. (p 70)

Ki-67 – A marker found in cells that are in the *growth fraction*. The growth fraction is the portion of cancer cells that are able to grow at any given time. A higher growth fraction indicates that the cancer is more dangerous. (p 79)

LCIS – See Lobular carcinoma *in situ*.

Leucopenia – Low levels of white blood cells in the blood. Makes a person susceptible to infection. *Febrile leucopenia*—fever because of a low white blood count—is a serious, life-threatening condition. (p 96)

LHRH agonist – A drug that stops the ovaries from making estrogens by blocking release of the hormone signals the brain normally uses to stimulate ovarian function. (p 97)

Liver function tests (LFTs) – Blood tests that look for evidence of liver or bone damage. When cancer grows in liver or bones, enzymes are spilled into the blood by damaged cells. LFTs look for increased levels of these enzymes, which indicate a possibility of cancer spread to bone or liver. (p 83)

Lobular carcinoma *in situ* (LCIS) – Also called lobular neoplasia. A finding on a pathology biopsy, LCIS indicates a higher risk of developing cancer in the future. This future cancer can be anywhere in either breast, unrelated to the location of the lobular carcinoma *in situ*. Some specialists believe it is better to call LCIS a "pre-cancer." (p 70)

Lobule/lobular – Lobules are the tiny milk-producing units at the ends of the ducts. Lobular refers to a type of invasive cancer thought to begin in the lobules. (p 71)

Lumpectomy – Originally used to describe removal of only the lump of a cancer from the breast, which is not an optimal treatment. Used colloquially to describe removal of the cancer without removing the breast. Removal of only the lump will usually leave positive margins and make recurrence likely. See wide local excision. (p 82 and 84).

Lymph – A water-and-protein mixture that collects as fluid in all parts of our body. Blood leaves the heart in arteries. It then passes through capillaries and returns to the heart in veins. All of the capillaries and small veins leak a small amount of fluid, which is called lymph. (p 88)

Lymphatics – Small, almost invisible, tubes that collect lymph and carry it back to the side of the neck, where the fluid is recycled into the blood. Lymphatics carry bacteria from an infection and debris from damaged cells and may carry cancer cells. (p 88)

Lymphedema – Swelling of a part of the body caused by damage of the lymphatics, which should drain lymph from that part of the body. In the context of breast cancer, this usually means swelling of the arm after surgery and/or radiation therapy have damaged lymphatics in the axilla. (p 90)

Lymph nodes – Virtual "filters" which pick up material carried in the lymphatics. Lymph nodes related to the breast may be an early site where invasive cancer cells begin their first metastases outside of the breast. They are not efficient filters in that they do not catch all cancer cells. (p 88)

Magnetic resonance imaging – Also called MRI. An imaging technique in which a person is exposed to an extremely strong magnet and pulses of radio waves that can be used by a computer to make images. Makes pictures without any radiation exposure. (p 36)

Malignant – A word to indicate that something is cancer and thus capable of causing major harm to a person. (p 64)

Mammogram – A specialized X-ray taken to focus on the breast with high-quality films, a machine used only for mammograms, and low doses of radiation exposure. (p 28)

Margins – The edge of the tissue removed at a biopsy, a partial mastectomy, or a mastectomy. For optimal control of cancer, the margin of tissue should not have cancer. For optimal assessment of margins, the pathologist should put special ink on the surface of the tissue to mark the edges before microscope slides are prepared. (p 85)

Marker - A laboratory test that provides information about a cancer, the risk of cancer, or another aspect of a person's health. (p 77

Mastectomy – An operation that removes the entire breast. Usually the nipple is removed if mastectomy is done for cancer unless the cancer is far away from the nipple. Muscles are not usually removed unless the cancer has grown directly into the muscles. (p 82 and 84)

Metabolic pathway – A set of genes and their proteins that collectively carry out some process in the life of cells. (p 102)

Metastasis/metastatic – Cancer that has grown outside of the breast area. Usually the lungs, liver, and bones are screened for metastases when invasive breast cancer is first diagnosed. (p 70 and 83)

Needle localization – A procedure in which the radiologist marks a place in the breast for biopsy by a surgeon. This procedure is used when the radiologist sees on the mammogram an area that is suspicious for cancer but cannot be felt on examination. (p 66)

Neoadjuvant therapy – Treatment with drugs given initially, before any surgery or radiation therapy. (p 87)

PALB2- A gene needed for *BRCA 1* and 2 to function. When *PALB2* has a mutation that makes it inactive, that causes *BRCA 1* and 2 to fail to prevent cancer just as though they were mutated. (p 43)

Partial mastectomy – see Wide Local excision

Pathological complete response (pCR)–Situation where neoadjuvant chemotherapy or hormone-based therapy was so successful that when the area where the cancer was located is removed, the pathologist cannot find any residual cancer in the specimen. (p 87)

Primary – A word used to indicate the place where a cancer starts, e.g., the primary site. (p 84)

Progesterone – A female hormone made primarily in the ovary and responsible for maturation of duct tissue. (p 51). Very strong progesterone-like drugs can treat breast cancer. (p 98)

Progesterone receptor (PR) – See Hormone receptors.

Prognosis – The expectations for the future of a patient. Prognosis is always a relative expectation. It is always based on experience with similar patients in the past. Prognosis is subject to individual variation. (p 17)

Prognostic score – A way of analyzing a cancer to determine how likely it is to spread to another part of the body. Indicates high or low risk independent of tumor size or node status. (p 81)

Prospective randomized trials - see Randomized trial

PubMed – http://www.ncbi.nlm.nih.gov/PubMed/ A free on-line service of the National Library of Medicine in which anyone can look up medical journal articles. It's free. It's your tax dollars at work!

Quadrantectomy (quadrectomy) – See Wide Local Excision

Radiation therapy – Use of high-energy radiation (like X-rays) to kill cancer cells. (p 92)

Randomized trial – A study of a treatment in which similar women are assigned randomly (by chance) to one treatment or another. The only recognized way to have a result that is free of bias created by the preconceived ideas of the persons testing a new or existing treatment. Since the women must be randomized before treatment, and such a study is done in a clinical setting with patients, it is sometimes called a prospective randomized clinical trial (p 19, 103)

Recurrence – Recurrence is when cancer grows another time after treatment of the initial primary cancer. (p 18, 70)

Relative risk – A term used to describe the relation between the occurrence of a cancer in one group and the occurrence of cancer in another group. May also describe the occurrence of events other than cancer. When relative risk is described in relative terms like twice, half, etc., it has an intuitive meaning with everyday usage of words. However, when expressed as a percentage, it can be confusing if one attempts to apply everyday meaning to the terms. For example, a risk of 4% in one group is twice the risk of 2% in another group. However, it is also correct to say that the relative risk of the first group is 2.0 or that the risk in the first group is 100% greater than in the second group. (p 40)

Risk Calculator - A computer program that combines many factors about a woman to estimate her risk of developing breast cancer over a period of time. (p 43)

Risk reduction – A term used to describe reduction in the risk of a bad event such as cancer recurrence or death. Like relative risk, it refers to a reduction of a portion of what the risk is before treatment begins. For example, if a therapy leads to a risk reduction of 25%, the absolute risk reduction is about one-quarter of the risk that existed before treatment. A risk of 40% before treatment becomes 30%, and a risk of 20% before treatment becomes 15%. (p 45, 47, 49)

SEER - Surveillance Epidemiology and End Results. A comprehensive database of population-based cancer information collected from cancer registries in the United States. SEER started with seven registries in 1973. There are now 20 tumor registries that contribute data to the SEER database.

Sentinel node – Like in the military term for a sentinel, the node that is most closely associated with a cancer. When the sentinel node contains cancer, there is higher risk of spread of cancer to other nodes and the body in general. When the sentinel node does not contain cancer (is negative) there is very low risk that cancer is in other nodes. (p 79)

Sonography – See ultrasound.

S-phase – The time during which an individual cell makes or synthesizes (hence the S) new chromosomes and DNA in preparation for dividing and becoming two cells. The higher the percentage of cells that are in S-phase, the more dangerous a cancer is. (p 81)

Stage – A term used to describe the location or locations of a breast cancer. Stage is a composite of the available information about the size of the primary cancer, whether cancer has metastasized to axillary lymph nodes, and whether there are metastases in other parts of the body. Higher stage is more dangerous. (p 77)

Statistics – The records of the events that have occurred in the lives of women who have had breast cancer in the past. Also refers to the mathematical tests used to determine if differences observed between groups happened by chance, or whether the differences observed between groups are likely to happen more than 95% of the time. (p 17)

Targeted biologic therapy – Use of antibodies or small molecules to stop or inhibit the action of one specific step in a metabolic pathway. (p 101)

Triple negative – A kind of breast cancer in which three main tests on a tumor (estrogen receptors, progesterone receptors, and HER2) are all negative. Triple negative is a simplified way to estimate whether a cancer has developed from basal cells. (p 80)

Triple test – A way to interpret the results of fine needle aspiration in conjunction with the results of mammograms and clinical breast examination. If all three tests indicate that an area is not cancer, there is a 99% probability that cancer is not present in that area. (p 65)

Ultrasound – Use of high-pitched sound waves to examine breast tissue. High-pitched sound waves bounce off solid tissues but not fluids. Can determine whether something is solid but cannot reliably exclude or diagnose cancer without a biopsy. No radiation exposure. (p 35)

Wide local excision – Removal of a cancer from the breast along with some apparently normal tissue around the cancer. The apparently normal tissue is removed because most invasive cancers have small projections of cancer into the surrounding, apparently normal tissue. If these "projections" are left in place, the cancer is likely to regrow. This is the method of surgery used for the NSABP (National Surgical Adjuvant Breast Project) and Milan trials for breastconserving therapy for early breast cancer. (p 82 and 84))

Wire localization – See Needle localization.

ACKNOWLEDGMENTS

I greatly appreciate those who helped make possible the Second Edition of It's your body...ASK. I thank Laurie King for thoughtful editing and content review, Polly Lockman for creative cover design and illustrations, Jim Shubin for excellent technical layout and production management - and on-the-fly editing in the process —and my family for their infinite support.

ABOUT THE AUTHOR

Dr. William H. Goodson III, is a graduate of Harvard Medical School and a recognized leader in breast cancer care. He practices as a physician and surgeon in San Francisco where he is also a Senior Scientist at California Pacific Medical Center Research Institute. He has written extensively on breast cancer and environmental causes of cancer, and his articles have appeared in such respected medical journals as Cancer (the scientific journal of the American Cancer Society), The American Journal of Medicine, Archives of Surgery, and the Oxford University Press journal, Carcinogenesis.

He has been a Professor of Surgery at the University of California, President of the San Francisco Medical Society, and Chairman of the Board of directors of the Institute for Medical Quality. He is a Fellow of The American College of Surgeons and member of the Society of University Surgeons, The Society for Surgical Oncology, The American Society for Clinical Oncology, and the American Society of Breast Surgeons.

Dr. Goodson was recognized with the Compassionate Caring Award from the Institute for Health and Healing, and he has been included in The Best Doctors in America for more than 25 years.

You can learn more about his practice at www.drwilliamgoodson.com .

CPSIA information can be obtained
at www.ICGtesting.com
Printed in the USA
FSOW03n1538060117
29176FS